READ THIS FIRST!

I hate writing introductions because I rarely read them. This is usually because the author tries to include some autobiographical anecdote about something that happened to him or her in childhood and quite frankly; I am just not interested. However, this is a "truth about" book in a series of them, so I try to pack it with important information from cover to cover.

I'm no doctor, nor do I have any kind of degree related to the subject matter of this book. As such you are welcome to judge me accordingly but, a whole lot of people have changed the world and the way you live and they did not have degrees either. So I recommend you read this booklet first, before you judge me and I think you will see that a person does not need a degree to be smart, hard working, well informed, and indeed an expert in their field.

That paragraph was lifted directly from the previous books in the series but I feel obligated to start by telling you the TRUTH about myself: I am NOT claiming to be some arrogant self-aggrandizing jackass with a wall full of diplomas. I am claiming to be a bewildered consumer like most people who just got tired of being so bewildered and went on a mission to find the TRUTH about nutrition (amongst many other topics for coming "truth about" books.)

One of the things that really got to me was the wide ocean of buzz words in the field of medicine and health. What is an antioxidant really? What does it do and why do I need them? For that matter what is fiber, what does it do and why do I need it? And so on.

Both of these come from plant foods and in fact there is a vast array of constituents in natural whole plant foods with names like flavinoids, phytosterols, etc, that are all members of the general classification of substances known as "The Phytonutrients" and this book is all about them. I even considered naming the book "The Truth About… Phytonutrients" but in the end I called it what I did because I thought it had a little more "sex appeal." So yes, I do want to sell books and I guess that makes me one of those money-grubbing monsters I keep calling out, but in all fairness I am no billionaire and have no such aspirations either. I write these books to help people. I know my cause is just and that is all that matters.

Mankind is primarily a plant eater. Over 90% of the daily food intake, on average, of modern indigenous tribes worldwide is comprised of plant foods. From this we deduce that throughout our evolutionary history going back hundreds of thousands to millions of years, we were essentially the same; hunter-gatherers who depended primarily on the gathering, not the hunting to find their daily sustenance.

Over those countless eons we evolved, adapted, continually changing and evolution will always follow the easiest, laziest pathways, the ones that most easily and efficiently solve the imperative problems; not the most difficult and complex possible solutions, but the simplest.

It is exactly because of this that we lost our ability to produce Vitamin C on our own. Why should our bodies continue to go through the effort to do this, wasting valuable resources and energy when all of the people are happily pigging out on oranges?

And it is also because of this laziness that we not only dropped making our own Vitamin C; our bodies became dependent not just on the fruits to provide Vitamin C, but on the entire package – the orange and all of its other constituents – as the delivery vehicle for that vitamin and we became just as dependent on those other things as we are for Vitamin C.

We did not evolve throughout all of those millennia boiling potatoes or beans either. That started much more recently within the last 15,000 to 35,000 years and we are still evolving, adapting, to this relatively new source of food, the SECONDARY FOODS that must be cooked in order to make them edible.

It was a huge technological innovation of the time. After we tamed fire primarily for warmth and light and to scare away predators in the night while we tried to get some sleep, someone accidentally left some meat next to the fire and when they ate it they found that it tasted pretty good. Later we would discover that by doing that, far fewer folks would get horribly sick and die (from the worms and bacteria in the meat.) And cooking was invented.

Eventually someone figured out that by boiling the tooth cracking seeds of the chick pea plant, they became soft and delicious and the technological revolution was born and we can imagine that our ancestors tried to boil everything in sight to see what would come out tasty and edible.

With this innovation, ancient man went from scavenging on a VERY SMALL percentage of raw edible plant species (a small fraction of one percent of all plants have raw edible parts) to being able to eat many more. The hunter-gatherers easily tripled their potential food sources over night.

This would lead to an instant population explosion and with it, many more smart folks walking around and that would lead to a better understanding of plants to the point where someone successfully grew them, rather than having to forage around for miles trying to find them, and civilization was born. Now we could stay in one place and raise the crops and the animals that would eat some of them and farming communities capable of easily feeding the masses grew into empires.

Why the story? The point is that these secondary foods were an amazing technological discovery for ancient man, but they are NOT PRIMARY foods. And even though we have over the ensuing millennia adapted to eating them, that process is still under way and not entirely complete. Evidence of this is plain and it is called "gluten intolerance" and "lactose intolerance" and the fact that beans cause… ahem, "digestive difficulties."

Now we are arrogant enough to believe that we can actually invent food from scratch despite the fact that our digestive tracts developed and adapted and evolved over hundreds of thousands of years to the raw edible plants that we ate that whole time and they are still only reluctantly adapting to all of those secondary foods that we already "invented" with the cooking process tens of thousands of years back.

I am very sure that in the early days of cooking that many people had severe digestive issues with those newly invented cooked foods. But back then the choices were severely limited; they either had to choke them down and suffer the gastrointestinal consequences or go without. And I have little doubt that some perished along the way because they simply couldn't eat the stuff at all. So the modern humans are the descendents of those who could manage to stomach those new foods. And in theory we could say that this process has begun once again with the new technological revolution of completely manufactured food.

But there is a big difference this time. We do NOT need this invented food in order to survive like our ancient ancestors did. Earth still provides enough for all 7 billion of us. We might be pushing the planet to its limits, but it can still support and feed everyone. Therefore no one NEEDS to eat artificial food and no one should because it is new to our digestive tracts and our bodies, and no creature adapts in a single life time; it takes many millennia and I do not want to be a new evolutionary dead end and drop dead because I am one of the current generation who cannot stomach the new foods.

But our problems are only beginning with the invention of fake foods like soda pop that has NOTHING THAT WAS EVER ALIVE IN IT. We are also becoming a sedentary society that works hard all day long by sitting in front of a computer in an air-conditioned cubicle. I am not criticizing it, just stating the fact. And humans were never meant to do that. We evolved over those hundreds of thousands of years foraging and hunting. We were made to toil not sit around all day.

And our technological world has brought us plenty of other poisons too like bleach fumes, gasoline fumes, radioactive fallout from nuclear bomb tests and the reactor disasters of Chernobyl and Fukushima. And of course the destruction of the majority of the ozone layer by hair sprays.

We sure do love to cobble up new chemicals and fancy machines and throw them around like there is no tomorrow. But there is a tomorrow and it always seems to bring us terrible news about the consequences of all of our fabulous creations.

The primary consequences of our actions are cancer and heart disease which are KILLING people by the hundreds of thousands each year. I would argue that many of those deaths are entirely PREVENTABLE too.

Right now one in three Americans will die of cancer, a disease that was one of the rarest known to medical science prior to World War II with only a handful - and I mean LESS THAN TEN – cases diagnosed by doctors each year. In the fifties these numbers exploded exponentially from hundreds per year to thousands to tens of thousands to hundreds of thousands of new cases each year. What changed? Two things: chemical additives to the foods we eat started appearing in the fifties and the nuclear bombs were set off in the mid-forties through the fifties. These bombs create what we all know very well as the mushroom cloud, this thing sends radioactive fallout as high as 30 miles, that's the edge of space, and the upper atmospheric winds can distribute that fallout worldwide and it only takes ONE RADIOACTIVE ATOM to be absorbed by you, to ultimately possibly cause cancer in you.

Although we can't go back in time and stop all of the deadly radioactive contamination caused by the nuclear bomb tests and the catastrophic reactor failures, contamination that IS killing people with cancer worldwide and will continue to do so for thousands of years into the future, we CAN do something about the foods we eat and we can start exercising which plays a critical role in human health.

I continually harp about changing to a diet consisting of nothing but natural whole foods and there is a reason for that: these are the foods that we EVOLVED eating. Our species adapted to these foods over hundreds of thousands of years and our digestive tracts are literally made to digest them and ONLY THEM and our bodies are made specifically to USE the vast array of molecules in them and they are NOT specifically designed to digest or use the constituents of TWINKIES, SODA POP or ROCKS (many minerals, if you have read Vol.3 – Minerals and the Other Essential Nutrients, are provided as the oxides which are essentially ROCKS.) And we are still in the midst of the process of adapting to the SECONDARY FOODS that must be cooked in order to become edible in the case of plant foods and most dairy products which were added to our menu after we settled down and started farming and being able to feed and raise livestock.

I am certain that almost every American who is not actively adding a solid well researched regimen of whole foods or natural supplements to their diet is MALNOURISHED. Three things are killing Americans:

1. They eat POISON in the form of CANCER CAUSING ADDITIVES to their PROCESSED foods on a DAILY BASIS. (And they are exposed to other POISONS also on a daily basis, like DIESEL ENGINE FUMES, HARSH CLEANER FUMES, etc.)
2. POOR DIET: even if you eat right, most of the plants are being grown in dead soil that has been overused for decades, the only reason the plants grow at all is because of the massive amounts of fertilizers being used on them – artificial, manufactured, chemical concoctions. This is what I affectionately call DIRTOPONICS. Just like HYDROPONICS or AEROPONICS, the plants must be given 100% of their nutritional requirements in order to grow, the only difference is that they are sitting in DEAD SOIL instead of pure water or air while they grow. Because of these conditions, many of the macro- and micro-minerals are dramatically reduced or completely missing, having been absorbed completely out of the soil by crops decades ago. Even the current crops, manage to eek out an existence based on their fertilizer sources of nutrients but cannot possibly be producing the supplements we expect from them in the quantities that they should have, hence we are all malnourished even if we eat the right foods because they simply no longer contain adequate, or natural, levels of the nutrients that they should be providing us.
3. LACK OF EXERCISE: You cannot expect to be healthy if all you do is sit in your car on the way to work. Sit at a desk all day at work, and sit at your TV all evening when you get home. You MUST find a way to do some aerobics, at least one hour DAILY.

This series was originally meant to guide you through the bewildering maze of the vitamin shelf at your favorite drug store but I have since decided to expand on that greatly and try to not only answer all of the questions like "What is fiber and what is it good for?" but to also cover the many curative/preventative natural products out there and to provide simple, quick solutions to the basics of how to live a healthy, happy and LONGER LIFE that is actually worth living.

These books are certainly not a substitute for professional advice. If you are currently on medication of any kind, you MUST CONSULT A DOCTOR before taking anything, including vitamins or any other supplements because they STRONGLY AFFECT the way your body works and can actually cause a VERY BAD REACTION in combination with certain strong medications.

Also, vitamins and minerals are ONLY THE BEGINNING; there are a multitude of ESSENTIAL NUTRIENTS that are neither vitamins nor minerals. Furthermore, MANY nutrients are NOT currently considered ESSENTIAL when they really ought to be and MOST of the phytonutrients that I cover in this book fall into this category.

Now, read and learn.

This is probably the number one item in our foods that we hear the most about that is not an actual essential nutrient. In fact, we probably hear far more about antioxidants than we do about any single essential nutrient except for perhaps the current hype around the Omega-3 fatty acids covered in Vol. 3.

So what are they and what do they do for us? This is an incredibly complicated question to answer, but I will try to "bottom-line it." Antioxidants basically neutralize negative ions in the body. Now, negative ions are everywhere, in fact the oxygen in the air we breath is a neutral molecule of two oxygen atoms bonded to each other called O_2, but these two atoms very easily separate and one of them will be an oxygen atom missing one electron and have a positive charge O^+ and the other will be an oxygen atom that stole the extra electron from the other one and it will be a negatively charged ion O^- and it is this one that allows fires to rage out of control and it is the one that hemoglobin grabs up in the lungs and delivers to all of the cells throughout the entire body to use to burn fuels that drive all of their metabolic functions including growth, maintenance, cell division and even the utilization of virtually all of the essential nutrients.

So the negatively charged oxygen ion is critical to practically all life on Earth. Only a handful of archaebacteria can live without it and we know them as anaerobic bacteria that thrive in the absence of oxygen and die off in its presence, because unless your biochemistry has been constructed around its usage, it is a deadly corrosive as dangerous as chlorine gas (the poisonous gas used during World War I that killed thousands of soldiers.) And because oxygen is the "poster child" of a powerful class of chemicals known as oxidants, they get their name from it.

Therefore oxygen is far from the only one that exists and cellular processes in the human body can release endless by-products and many of these chemical waste compounds are, you guessed it, oxidants or atoms or molecules that have a high tendency to gain an electron and become oxidants which are very damaging and corrosive materials that can and will damage healthy cells and one of the very worst possible forms of damage to any living cell in the human body is if the DNA in the nucleus gets corrupted.

Most of the time, the damaged cell simply dies and gets dissolved and delivered to the intestines and/or the kidneys for removal, but sometimes that damaged DNA can lead to a cell that has lost the blueprint of the organ that it is a part of and it begins to divide and grow and all of its damaged children continue to do this and form a tumor, growing beyond the design of the organ because they lost the DNA map and don't know what they are doing any more.

Most of the time this damaged cell is detected by the immune system and the white blood cells attack and destroy it and send the rubble through the blood for the intestines and the kidneys to clean out and dump. But on rare occasions, the damaged cell manages to go unnoticed and continues to divide and 2 become 4 become 8 and pretty soon you have a tumor.

One of the best ways to prevent this whole mess from getting started in the first place is to equip the cells with large amounts of substances that are designed specifically to neutralize those oxidants when they form. If that is done, then those dangerous negative ions can't do any damage and the whole calamity can be averted before it ever gets started. Those are the antioxidants.

So all of the cells in the human body are constantly working, burning sugar with oxygen to create the energy they need to stitch together a single amino acid molecule or to stitch that to another one as they build their proteins. This is even taking place all through the night while we sleep. So while our brain unwinds, practically every cell in the body including those in the brain are burning through sugar and building things and creating waste by-products including a large number of oxidants that are expelled by the cells into the blood stream and make their way to the intestines and the kidneys for removal.

Because our cells are filled with tiny delicate molecular structures including and in particular their DNA, these dangerous substances must be neutralized as quickly as possible and as often as possible, right there inside of the cells. And this can happen because there are many antioxidants that the cells will absorb and use for many different intracellular processes and if there is an abundance of these molecules around, then most of the potentially dangerous waste by-products will get neutralized if they misbehave and absorb an extra electron and become dangerous oxidants.

One of the very best antioxidants you can give to your cells is VITAMIN C. Virtually every cell in the human body uses it for intracellular processes and in abundance it works like a protective blanket within the cell to quickly neutralize any dangerous oxidant that shows up. Vitamin C is water soluble and can be taken in extreme excesses with no harmful side effects and since all of the cells in the body need it and will take it in, then large amounts of this powerful antioxidant can go a long way to preventing the build up and damage caused by all of those waste by-product oxidants that all of the cells in the body are making all day and night every day of our lives from the skin to the bones and everything in between.

Vitamin E is another powerful antioxidant and one of its primary functions within all cells in the human body is to prevent damage and corruption to the DNA in the nucleus of the cell. One way it does this is simply because it is an antioxidant and so it can neutralize any stray oxidant molecules wandering around in the nucleus of the cell. Vitamin E is an oil soluble vitamin and should be kept below 250% of the RDA on a daily basis which is of little concern to most Americans who by and large are suffering from chronic Vitamin E deficiency because it is almost only found in seeds and nuts which most of us normally do not eat daily. And I believe that this is one of the major causes of EPIDEMIC CANCER in our society today.

And because antioxidants prevent DNA damage and promote longer and stronger life for each and every single cell in the body, antioxidants promote better cellular function and less cell death which means the organs all function better, this reduces stress on the intestines and kidneys to remove dangerous waste by-products and dissolved dead cell matter, and of course the antioxidants help prevent DNA damage that can result in a cancerous cell. The end result is better overall health, less overall organ degeneration (works like anti-aging) and helps prevent cancer. Who doesn't want to live a LONGER, HEALTHIER, CANCER-FREE LIFE?

But the story of the antioxidants has only just begun. You see, the immune system uses oxidants (not antioxidants) to ward off viruses in particular. These nasty things are sometimes little more than wandering strands of DNA that attempt to invade the cell and usurp the DNA replication machinery in the nucleus and try to fool that machinery into making more of them instead. Some oxidants in the bloodstream and within the cell are there by design to bond with those foreign DNA strands and neutralize them – they basically are there to purposely damage those DNA strands because they are unwanted.

To that end many folks have erroneously argued that an excess of antioxidants could, in theory, suppress the immune system or disrupt these functions and allow viruses to run rampant. Obviously more research is required on the subject but suffice it to say that an extra dose of antioxidants provided by natural whole foods – and they are almost only found in plant foods by the way, like oranges, or kiwis, is NOT going to make you susceptible to the flu. It is going to help you fight it off mainly because the immune system will not be so busy trying to deal with all of those stray waste by-product oxidants running around inside of you. In other words, some of the purposely built oxidants might get neutralized by extreme excesses of antioxidants, but the immune system is perfectly capable of monitoring their levels and making more as needed.

The bottom line is that antioxidants are the ultimate detoxifiers in the bloodstream and within the cells and if you are not all clogged up with your own waste by-product toxins, and healthier in general, then your immune system has less to worry about and it will be stronger too. And don't forget that Vitamin C and E and most of the other antioxidants in the whole natural foods that we eat do more than just act like antioxidants, they are involved in the intracellular machinery in specific biochemical roles that the cells need. So don't be shy, load up on those antioxidants!

One last point of interest; antioxidants aside from playing multiple roles in cellular processes also have different "affinities" too. This means that some of them are good at neutralizing straight negative oxygen ions while others are good at neutralizing hydroxyl (–O-H) groups. Some grab on tightly while others grab on loosely and some can neutralize only a few radicals while others can neutralize huge quantities of them.

Obviously antioxidants are an enormous group of compounds with representatives in most phytonutrient chemical classes, and each has a different affinity and strength as an antioxidant. The Oxygen Radical Absorption Capacity or ORAC score was developed to be able to compare the various antioxidants against each other and to evaluate which foods were the best in terms of their antioxidant content. The score is based on the antioxidative power of 100 grams (about 3.5 oz,) of each food.

So, the higher the score, the more antioxidant power the food has. However, we must keep in mind that each antioxidant has its own affinity (the things it likes to neutralize best) as well as its other roles in cellular metabolism. As such, Vitamin E has critical functions in the protection of DNA during cell division and so it is mostly found in the nucleus of our cells. Others play an active and powerful role as antioxidants while traveling through the bloodstream where some assist the red blood cells, and so on. So while the "raw" ORAC score can tell you which foods are loaded with powerful antioxidants, it does not tell us which specific antioxidants are present in the food and where they perform their antioxidative roles within the human body or what other functions they get involved in either.

Nevertheless it is good to know what foods have very high ORAC scores and try to incorporate them into your daily diet. Some typical foods loaded with antioxidants of excellent power are tomatoes which are loaded with lycopene which is about 150 TIMES more potent than Vitamin C as an antioxidant: ORAC score of about 500. Carrots, loaded with beta-carotene of similar strength to lycopene (the two are in fact related which I will discuss in an upcoming chapter,) have an ORAC score of about the same. However, dark chocolate (100% Pure cacao) has an ORAC score of over 20,000! So 5 oz. of pure dark chocolate has FORTY TIMES more antioxidant power than 5 oz. of carrots! Just remember that the carrots are loaded with beta-carotene which your body can easily convert into Vitamin A which you MUST have in adequate supplies on a daily basis. So it is not about substituting perceived bad foods for good ones, it is about ADDING better and better foods to a daily eating regimen that consists of nothing but good foods. Incidentally, cloves have one of the highest ORAC scores of any commonly available food: over 300,000! But who in their right mind is going to eat 5 ounces of that!

Still it doesn't change the fact that most of the spices including oregano, rosemary, cilantro, etc. all have fantastically high ORAC scores and you should make every effort to use them in your natural whole foods cooking and I dump them liberally into my oil and vinegar salad dressing too.[42] (Sorry about the order of the end note references, it was actually the content of the book that got rearranged at the last minute.)

END OF CHAPTER QUIZ
1. Antioxidants neutralize:
   A. Negative ions
   B. Oxidants
   C. Waste metabolic by-products
   D. All of the above
   Answer D; All of the above describe the same things; substances that build up in the cells that can damage their delicate molecular machinery including DNA.
2. Cancer is basically:
   A. Any cells that keep dividing out of control.
   B. The result of damaged or corrupted DNA in a cell.
   C. Both A and B
   D. Neither A or B
   Answer: C. Cancer is caused by damage to the DNA which leads to out-of-control cellular division and growth.
3. Two powerful and essential nutrients that can greatly assist in the prevention of cancer are also antioxidants and they are:
   A. Vitamin C
   B. Vitamin E
   C. Both A and B
   D. Neither A or B.
   Answer: C. Both Vitamin C and E are used by all cells in the body and an abundant supply of them can definitely help prevent cancer.
4. The body uses oxidants to:
   A. Aid in digestion
   B. Aid the immune system
   C. Aid the function of antioxidants
   D. The body does not use oxidants
   Answer: B. The immune system uses oxidants to neutralize invading viruses by damaging them and rendering them harmless. The problem is that a build up of unwanted waste by-product oxidants could damage our own DNA in our own cells and possibly cause those cells to turn cancerous.

This is another health food buzz word for the past several decades and I never knew what this stuff was or what it was good for until I went through the trouble of studying up on it.

Fiber is, by definition, found only in plants. It is the fraction of the total plant food mass that cannot be digested or broken up and absorbed by the intestines. Since almost all of the meat and fat in an animal food portion is pure CP (Complete Protein) and the fat is pure high density carbohydrate fuel (higher density than even sugar,) we can and do successfully absorb almost all of the animal meat portions that we eat. Of course, I am talking about the foods in the coolers in the "Meat and Dairy" section of your grocery store like ground beef, steak, pork chops, chicken wings, etc. And I am not talking about the stranger possible animal food items. (We will just leave it at that!)

As expected, those foods highest in fiber content as a percentage of the total mass of the serving are SECONDARY plant foods; those that must be cooked in order to become edible. In other words, before you cooked the food, it was inedible and therefore MOST of it was basically fiber. The cooking process begins to break down the tough bonds in the plant mass which is why potatoes change from being crisp to being mushy. In the process, the smaller molecules (the broken up pieces of the large ones that had the tough bonds) are more readily digestible and thus the inedible food is transformed into an edible one.

This process was a boon to early man because with its discovery the number of edible plants available in the surrounding environment swelled and gave early mankind far more food than was available to his ancestors. Think about this: far less than one percent of ALL species of plants on Earth have edible parts for human consumption including the SECONDARY food plants that must be cooked in order to be rendered edible. The very best way to see this is in any of the wilderness survival shows on TV. I have seen survivalists dropped into the middle of dense equatorial jungles where they are literally surrounded by vegetation and during their excursion they are starving and desperate to find food.

So the accidental discovery of cooking made it possible for humans to find more food which in turn led to the ability to feed more people which in turn led to population increases: more people, more children and a higher survival rate of the species. You might say that survival throughout human history has always centered primarily on finding food, not fighting off big predators – not that they are of zero significance, just relatively low on the scale of important problems to be solved and cooking secondary foods that transformed them from inedible into edible foods was a significant triumph in human innovation and marked the beginning not only of our rise to our current state of prominence, but also marked the beginning of civilization itself.

I always advise people to cut way back on the secondary foods as a category; far less grains of any kind, far less roots like potatoes that must be cooked in order to become edible, and ZERO BEANS. Even though there are several different kinds of beans that have some nutritional value once cooked, the fact of the matter is that for the most part these things are not very healthy especially when they become the majority of the total food mass that a person consumes on a daily basis. We all know the joke about eating too many beans, that they give you gas, and there is a reason for that: they are trouble for the digestion even after they have been soaked for hours and boiled for hours. All that means is that a VERY INEDIBLE FOOD has been beaten down to the point that it is now MARGINALLY EDIBLE. But they still give the digestive tract a hard time and should be avoided.

And the last major member of the secondary foods list is legumes. These too are somewhat problematic for the same reason: a totally inedible food has been beaten down by the cooking process in order to become edible. However, the difference is that the legumes are somewhat different. And these particular seeds are loaded with nutrients. The main bulk of the entire seed is in fact a nugget of high density organic nutrients for the plant embryo to begin growing and be able to break out of the seed shell. As such legumes are rich in many significant essential nutrients especially the minerals which no organism on Earth can manufacture: they MUST BE FOUND either in the soil, in the case of plants, or the food in the case of animals. This is very different from organic molecules, simply constructed from the basic organic chemistry elements of Carbon, Hydrogen, Oxygen and Nitrogen: what I call CHON molecules. Amino aids and therefore proteins are mostly constructed from these but many do have other elements in them like sulfur and phosphorus. But straight up CHON molecules can be built from any other CHON molecules that happen to be around, so many organisms can use what's already available – the entire organism is basically constructed out of CHON molecules – and can make rearrangements to its heart's content. These are not nearly as difficult to deal with, because they can be manufactured from others in the body, but the minerals cannot be manufactured by any organism because we do not contain nuclear synthesis reactors that can change one element into another; only the stars (and nuclear reactors and bombs) can do that.

So legumes like green peas and chick peas and peanuts, now and then, making up a small minority of the mass of your diet, are not just acceptable, they are recommended and may be the only way some people can get the vital minerals their bodies need.

The bottom line here is that these secondary foods including the grains, roots, and legumes in particular are all loaded with fiber because they are overloaded with it (before we cook them) to the point that raw they are inedible because of all of that fiber in their composition. Remember that "fiber" does not mean one specific molecule, but instead a class of molecules and there are a lot of them. Cellulose in its various and sundry forms is a fine example of fiber and it is completely inedible. Grass has so much cellulose in it that you could cook it for weeks until it completely dissolves and it would STILL BE INEDIBLE because the molecules have been reduced dramatically in size, but they are still fiber and still impossible to digest.

So while we all know that we should leave the grass to the cows and the goats, the point is that virtually all plants contain fiber. They use these molecules to build their cell walls to strengthen their stems and leaves so that they can stand up straight (I am speaking primarily of the "herbaceous" plants, little green stemmed plants that do not use WOOD for this structural support.) And a diet based on natural whole foods with the predominant mass consisting of plant foods, must be high in fiber right? Not necessarily so.

You see raw broccoli is very stiff and crunchy, but boil it for 20 minutes and it is very soft and mushy. The fiber is still there but some of it has been reduced to smaller molecules by the cooking process and so some of the fiber has been lost. This varies from one plant to the next, some may lose a small amount while others may lose most of it. And some plants start with much lower amounts than others even raw. What we need is food sources that have a high PERCENTAGE of fiber in them at the time of consumption. And this is exactly why I encourage folks who want to have the healthiest diet possible, to eat RAW EDIBLE PLANT foods as the primary bulk of their whole natural foods diet.

Even though we have been cooking for something like 15,000 to 35,000 years as a species, we spent about 2 MILLION years prior to that eating nothing but raw edible plant foods as the main course of our daily diet as hunter-gatherers and that is what our digestive tracts are MADE FOR: those are the foods that our digestive system is specifically designed to digest and get the majority of our nutrients from (ends in a preposition, I know.) In other words, we NEED all of that fiber even though we don't actually digest any of it.

So if we do not digest it, then what do we need it for (can a question end in a preposition)? It plays a critical role in the health of the inner lining of our intestines. Remember that as a species we have spent over a million years evolving up to where we are now; eating these raw edible plant foods. So we have adapted to not just be able to tolerate the percentage of the mass that cannot be digested, but to also depend on it to be there. People who have very low fiber diets for decades throughout their lives are much more susceptible to a wide assortment of digestive tract maladies including cancer itself.

But fiber also plays a role in reducing cholesterol and other functions that at first would seem impossible. How can something that travels all the way through my digestive tract reduce the cholesterol in my body? Plant fiber – and there are two kinds, water soluble and water-insoluble – can cling to cholesterol molecules and carry them all the way through the digestive tract and keep it from being absorbed by the intestinal lining as well as serve as sort of a cleaning brush for all of those microscopic finger-like protrusions in the intestinal lining that do all of the absorbing of nutrients and releasing of biological waste products of the body. Remember that this is an adaptation that started way back in the deep, dark, unknown evolutionary beginning and it has been honed over time to become very efficient and very reliable and we are very dependent on it in order to maintain optimal health.[43]

The one grain food that I do recommend highly is oatmeal (real old-fashioned and NOT instant) and I eat it most days for breakfast and so should you. It is well known as a "heart health" food and the reason is that it is so high in fiber as a percentage of the mass of the oatmeal and that is an excellent way to start your day (and start your digestive process of the day is what I really mean.) It is also loaded with molybdenum which we use to make Molybdenum Cofactor or MOCO. If you do not have molybdenum, and therefore no MOCO, then you cannot efficiently and properly manipulate various sulfur containing compounds in your body and those are involved in some of the amino acids. No new amino acids means no new proteins which means no new cells and you start to degenerate; you age faster, all organ systems suffer, and you will be sickly and die earlier than you should have. Oatmeal gives you a tremendous two for one: very high in fiber and all the molybdenum your body needs to properly work with sulfur. Crisp raw edible plant matter like a big tossed salad for lunch will continue the process of giving your body lots of additional fiber and plenty of essential nutrients as well. Later I will discuss more high fiber foods, but as long as you stick to these two you are well on your way to taking care of your fiber intake needs and thus taking care of your digestive tract health for a longer better life.[51]

END OF CHAPTER QUIZ
1. Fiber is:
    A. The contents of the food that cannot be digested.
    B. Found almost exclusively in plants
    C. A whole enormous class of different molecules
    D. All of the above.

Answer: D. Fiber is a huge class of molecules found in almost all plant foods exclusively that is matter within them that cannot be digested.

2. The foods highest in fiber are:
    A. Secondary foods like grains and legumes
    B. Raw edible foods like spinach and apples
    C. Both A and B
    D. Neither A or B

Answer: C. Both secondary foods that must be cooked in order to become edible and raw edible foods eaten raw are the best sources of fiber.

3. The major function of fiber is:
    A. Aids digestion by physically scrubbing the intestinal lining
    B. Providing additional calories
    C. Providing nutrients for heart health
    D. Reduces cholesterol

Answer: A. This is the primary function of fiber although it does bind to cholesterol reducing its ability to be absorbed which promotes heart health. Fiber itself cannot be digested so it provides no calories or nutrients at all.

4. Which of the following can help prevent cancer?
    A. Eliminating processed and packaged foods high in chemical additives.
    B. Switching to an all-natural whole foods diet high in fiber and antioxidants
    C. Getting ALL 41 essential nutrients in sufficient quantities in natural whole foods daily.
    D. All of the above.

Answer: D. The only thing missing is exercise and you will be on the way to avoiding this dreadful disease.

5. The ONE food loaded with molybdenum that is necessary for proper utilization of sulfur in our foods Is:
    A. Broccoli
    B. Grape juice
    C. Dark chocolate
    D. Oatmeal

Answer: D. Oatmeal. This is the only readily available food that has MANY good nutrients for the body as well as plenty of fiber and it is also packed with Molybdenum which allows us to metabolize sulfur.

This is another health industry buzz word of late and it refers to all of the other organic molecules in the foods we eat other than fiber (which is another huge class of organic molecules in the foods we eat that cannot be digested or absorbed by the digestive tract,) carbohydrates and proteins. However, "phyto" means plant, so "phytonutrients" is referring to all of the other natural organic compounds found in plant foods that are also digestible and absorbable by the digestive tract.

And there are literally countless thousands of them that we have identified and those that we have identified are only the tip of the iceberg: we have likely only identified about 0.1% of them all, and very few have been well researched as to their effects on the human body. Therefore it is likely that science will not identify all of these compounds by the end of the 21st century and very likely will not be able to do all of the research on all of those compounds to know exactly what they do for us either.

But the fact that these compounds exist is undeniable and the fact that we need them is equally undeniable. As we discover the chemical formula of each one and then subject it to rigorous clinical testing we then discover that each one invariably plays a crucial role in human health. So they are out there in all of those plant foods and many of them play not only critical daily nutrition roles but also curative/preventative roles as well.

I will list the kinds or classes of phytonutrients, but we have identified many individual compounds within each of these classes and some classes may contain literally tens of thousands to millions of different individual compounds. Some of these unique compounds have unique roles that no other compound in that class does which makes the whole thing even more complicated. But there is no reason to throw our hands up in the air either; all you have to do is make sure that along with the superfoods that guarantee that we are getting our daily requirements of the known 41 essential nutrients, that you also scatter in as many different whole natural foods as you can – variety is the key because somewhere in one of those foods you add to your natural whole foods regimen will be a vital compound that your body needs and by rotating through many different natural foods you will make sure that you get it at least every so often which is far better than going without until you break down because of a chronic lack of it.

THE LIST OF PHYTONUTRIENTS

1) **TERPENOIDS** – This is a huge class of compounds with many different classes of compounds that fall into it including:

    A) **CAROTENOIDS** – Also called "tetraterpenes" are built from 8 molecules called isoprenes each being a chain of 5 carbon atoms, so the carotenoids all have 40 carbon atoms in a specific arrangement in them. There are two major subclasses: the carotenes and the xanthophylls and there are about 1,100 identified carotenoids to date. The carotenoids are responsible for the bright reds, oranges, and yellows in many plants including daffodils and the fall colors of many deciduous trees' leaves in autumn like maple as well as the red color of tomatoes, the orange color of carrots, and the yellow color of squash. Many are key nutrients to the human body including beta-carotene which is the antioxidant precursor to Vitamin A (that the body can use and transform into Vitamin A as needed) found in carrots and mentioned in Vol.2 – Vitamins, as well as LYCOPENE, ZEAXANTHIN and LUTEIN which I cover in an upcoming chapter.[1]

B) **TRITERPENOIDS** – Another large class of compounds built around 6 isoprene groups and thus have 30 carbon atoms in them. Most are pure hydrocarbons with no other atoms in them other than the 30 carbons and 48 hydrogen atoms. All plants and animals make triterpenes including squalene which is the precursor to all steroids. About 200 distinct carbon-hydrogen arrangements have been identified thus far and a later chapter will discuss the SAPONINS found in many edible plants.[5]

C) **DITERPENOIDS** – Based on four isoprene groups these molecules are built around a specific kind of arrangement of 20 carbon atoms and you have certainly heard about one of these called retinol – a.k.a. VITAMIN A. And while the rest of the group may not be as critical to human health as retinol, there is no question that the group is under investigation because many diterpenes have antimicrobial and anti-inflammatory effects.[10]

D) **MONOTERPENOIDS** – These are mostly pure hydrocarbons built on two isoprenes and thus have 10 carbons and 16 hydrogen atoms in them. D-limonene is derived from citrus peels and added to products to give them either the aroma and/or flavor of oranges or citrus.[11]

E) **PHYTOSTEROLS** – This is another major class of plant compounds that are basically any of the above terpenoids (tetra-, tri-, di- or monoterpenoids) in which at least one of the hydrogen atoms has been replaced by an –O-H group turning it into an organic alcohol. Over 200 plant sterols have already been identified and they are actually similar in construction to cholesterol. Plant sterols have been offered as supplements for the reduction of cholesterol for years although there is currently no evidence that they are effective in this role. But chances are that you have heard of at least one phytosterol: alpha-tocopherol a.k.a. VITAMIN E.[13]

2) **PHENOLICS** – This is another major class of plant compounds with many large subclasses under it including:

A) **MONOPHENOLS** – Many of these are found in spices and have antiseptic (antibacterial) as well as systemic effects (work in various roles throughout the human body.)[15] Apiole found in celery and parsley was used in the past to treat menstrual problems and carvacrol is the characteristic pungent aroma of oregano and has been shown to kill many species of oral bacteria associated with tooth decay and possibly gum disease. So start adding plenty of oregano to your recipes, its good for killing those nasty bacteria in your mouth![16][44]

B) **POLYPHENOLS** – This is another very large class of compounds and very little study has been done on them as a group mainly because there are so many of them. They are found in most edible plants from apples to zucchini and tannic acid – the bitter dark brown astringent in tea – is a derivative of tannins, another large group of polyphenolic compounds.

C) **FLAVONOIDS** – This is a subcategory of the phenolics and contains over FIVE THOUSAND identified compounds so far. To say that these compounds are ubiquitous in plant foods would be an understatement. And there are three major subcategories of them as well including: ISOFLAVONOIDS of which there are six subcategories: flavones, flavonols, flavanones, flavanonols, flavans, and flavan-3-ols, AURONES, and ANTHOCYANIDINS. I'll mention a few of the individual compounds in an upcoming chapter.[17]

D) **CHALCANOIDS** – All chalcanoids share a similar basic structure involving two benzyl rings connected by a carbon chain of three atoms one of which has a double bonded oxygen attached to it. That =O group sticking out of the carbon chain between the two benzene rings in the molecular structure makes the chalcanoids ketones by definition.

WHAT IS A BENZYL GROUP?

This is the now classic benzene ring of six carbon atoms first correctly identified by Kekule while trying to figure out how a hydrocarbon like benzene could consist of 6 carbon atoms and 6 hydrogen atoms (impossible in any straight or branched chain, by the way.) And it looks like this:

```
              H       H
              |       |
              C   =   C
             /         \
          H-C           C-H
            \\         //
              C   -   C
              |       |
              H       H
```

This ring is usually just represented as a hexagon and is understood to include the six carbons and the hydrogen atom attached to each one. Only when the hydrogen is replaced by something else is the replacement atom or group drawn into the molecular diagram. The confusing thing about these rings is that they go by many different names including: phenyl, aryl, benzyl, benzene ring and aromatic ring but all of these names mean the same thing.

Chalconoids are mainly intermediary compounds found in virtually all plants and are used to make other compounds like many flavonoids. However, there is a lot of interest in these compounds because they show an array of interesting effects including: antibacterial, antifungal, anti-inflammatory and ANTITUMOR properties and they are currently under investigation.[52]

E) **FLAVONOLIGNANS** – These compounds are part flavonoid and part lignan and you have heard of at least one significant member of this rather rare group: silymarin found in Milk Thistle which serves as a liver tonic to promote liver health and repair.[53]

F) **LIGNANS** – Originally associated with wood (lignum is Latin for wood) lignans have been found in almost all plants and our intestinal bacteria transform plant lignans into animal lignans that we use. The category is quite large and any diet consisting of whole natural foods will provide you with plenty of them.[54]

G) **PHYTOESTROGENS** – These interesting compounds are chemically similar to estrogen produced in all mammals and it is believed that certain plants make them in large quantities as a defensive mechanism aimed at grazing animals. By pumping them full of "fake" estrogen, they decrease the fertility of the grazing flock which means there will be fewer mouths to feed over time allowing the plants to continue to proliferate. We do readily absorb phytoestrogens from the foods we eat and all research to date has been inconclusive concerning human fertility rates and while most scientists consider claims that phytoestrogens promote cardiovascular, metabolic, and central nervous system health are at best anecdotal, these benefits have not been properly tested in clinical trials either. So for now, there is no way to know for sure.[23]

H) **STILBENOIDS** – These are similar in structure to the chalcanoids but the two benzyl rings are connected by a chain of two carbon atoms instead of three and there is no double bonded oxygen atom present. Instead there are two –O-H groups attached to the benzyl rings making them phenolic (the term means "contains benzyl rings") alcohols. These too are precursors to the synthesis of other organic molecules but many are produced in significant quantities in certain plants for their antifungal properties. Stilbenoids are also powerful antioxidants and you might have heard of one of them: resveratrol being offered as a supplement making many health claims, possibly true since it is an antioxidant.[55]

I) **CURCUMINOIDS** – These consist of the two benzyl rings connected by a chain of seven carbon atoms hence the chemical name diarylheptanoids (di- meaning two, -aryl- refers to the benzyl rings, -heptan- refers to a carbon chain of seven atoms.) The group is however named after the first and most well known member of the group: curcumin, the bright yellow substance in the spice turmeric. Scientists question its efficacy as an antimutagen (prevents and even fights existing cancer) but there is a substantial amount of anecdotal evidence that suggests that it might have some positive effects, The problem with curcumin and the some of the other curcuminoids is that it transforms from one form to another depending on whether it is dissolved in water or a nonpolar organic solvent. In the organic solvents the seven carbon chain has a ketone group (double bonded oxygen) and an alcohol group (–O-H group) attached to it. In water the alcohol group drops the extra hydrogen and becomes another =O or ketone group. This inherent instability makes the compound difficult to test and confirm its efficacy and because it is impossible to verify its chemical structure, it is impossible to synthesize and use as a patented drug as well. But we have no interest in whether the money-grubbers can make a profit with it, we are only interested in its power to promote better health.[26][56]

J) **TANNINS** – This vast group includes the subcategories: tannins, hydrolysable tannins, condensed tannins, phlorotannins, and flavono-ellagitannins. These molecules are found in most plants and are called polyphenolic meaning they have many benzyl rings in them. Some subcategories have molecular weights ranging from about 500 to 3000 (each carbon atom has a molecular weight of 12 and each hydrogen has a molecular weight of 1, so these are huge molecules) while others have molecular weights of over 20,000. Tannins bind to proteins and amino acids and were originally used in tanning animal hides into leather because they remove the proteins and amino acids and they cause the dry puckering mouth sensation caused by unripe fruit. Hydrolysable tannins are found in most teas and berries.[27]

K) **AROMATIC ACIDS** – This is another huge group divided into the two subcategories: phenolic acids and hydroxy-cinnamic acids. Salicylic acid (aspirin) was discovered from the chemical analysis of willow bark tea used by Native Americans for pain relief. But it is also found in trace amounts in many common foods. Vanillic acid is found in vanilla beans and natural vanilla extract. Amongst the hydroxycinnamic acids, cinnamic acid is found in cinnamon but also in aloe vera, and coumarin creates the distinctive smell of freshly mowed grass but is also found in some fruits. Many of these natural acids have been used in traditional therapies including aromatherapy for thousands of years.[28][29]

L) **PHENYLETHANOIDS** – This rather small group of phenolic compounds has an array of them present in olive oil including Tyrosol, Hydroxytyrosol, Oleocanthal, and Oleuropein making olive oil of particular interest although there has been little research done thus far.[60]

M) **UNCATEGORIZED PHENOLICS** – It should come as no surprise that this is by far the largest group primarily because "anything goes" in the way of molecular structure and the vast majority of all plant compounds likely fall into this relatively unexplored realm of phytochemistry. Notable molecules that do not fall into any other category include capsaicin, the "heat" in the hot peppers, gingerol, the strong aroma and flavor of ginger, and a group called the alkylresorcinols found in many whole grains.[30][31][50]

3) **GLUCOSINOLATES** – These comprise another major category of phytochemicals and their key feature is that they have sulfur in them and include the following subcategories:

A) **ISOTHIOCYANATE PRECURSORS** – A notable compound in this group is sinigrin although there are many others.

B) **AGLYCONES** – These include the subcategories: dithiolthiones, organosulfides, and the indoles. The above isothiocyanate precursors are used to make the dithiolthiones. Sulfur may not be considered an essential nutrient by the FDA (in that they have not established an RDA – Recommended Daily Allowance – for it,) but it is necessary to ALL LIFE on Earth because it is found in some amino acids including methionine, one of the NINE ESSENTIAL amino acids that must be in the foods we eat, as well as several others like cysteine which our cells can make themselves presumably from the other compounds like these that are prevalent in certain foods. The indoles are a gigantic group of molecules with a vast array of functions in plants and are also common in fungi. Notable compounds are Indole-3-carbinol found in many common vegetables, Allicin and Alliin found in garlic, as well as Allyl isothiocyanate, Piperine and Syn-propanethial-S-oxide all of which are found in common available foods that most people eat.[32]

4) **BETALAINS** – This is another distinct and small group of phytochemicals found in high concentrations in Beets and that we know very little about thus far.[35]

5) **CHLOROPHYLLS** – We all know what chlorophyll is; the green coloring of all green plants and it is the molecule that captures light

from the sun and frees an electron that can do the work of constructing sugar, the energy from which is then used to construct all of the other molecules that make up the plant, by the way. But there are a few forms of chlorophyll and they all contain a magnesium atom and magnesium is one of the essential nutrients that we need to build enzymes and we need a lot of it on a daily basis. It is present in virtually all edible plant leaves even those that are not green like red cabbage.[37]

6) **UNCATEGORIZED ORGANIC ACIDS** – This is another potentially enormous group of molecules of which we have only begun to scratch the surface. Notable organic acids that fall into this group include many different acids that contribute to the flavors of the foods, but may have other far more significant roles in the human body as well.

7) **AMINES** – Also a vast and relatively unexplored group of molecules mainly because of their numbers and similarity to most of the other groups. These all contain a nitrogen atom from which they get their name. Many of these when converted into an acid by adding an –O-O-H group to them become the very well known AMINo acids. You know enough chemistry now to realize that phenylalanine, one of the NINE ESSENTIAL amino acids, is an amine (ends in –ine denoting a nitrogen compound) an organic acid containing the –O-O-H group and it has a benzyl ring in it somewhere (because of the phenyl- in the name.)[57]

8) **CARBOHYDRATES** – This is an incredibly large group of organic compounds in fact most of the above could be considered carbohydrates in the broadest sense; chemicals that contain carbon, hydrogen and oxygen in them. But in the strictest sense these refer to a specific arrangement and ratio of carbon to hydrogen to oxygen and include the monosaccharides (simple sugars) and polysaccharides (two or more sugar molecules bonded together) including starches and even cellulose.[58]

9) **PROTEASE INHIBITORS** – This is a very interesting group of compounds of enormous molecular size and complexity that work to inhibit proteases which are the compounds that break down proteins. While we might think protease inhibitors are a good thing, they really aren't. Our cells need to break down proteins all the time. But deficiency in at least one such protease inhibitor called A1AT can lead to disease. It is currently not clear if these compounds would be effective at reducing unnecessary levels of protein breakdown in the human body in such roles as anti-aging, because our cells often need to break down proteins. Since these are such large molecules it is unlikely that they would survive our digestive process intact.[59]

(This list and most of the information included was obtained from www.wikipedia.org.)[33]

WHAT DOES ALL OF THAT REALLY MEAN?

Well it certainly was a lot more chemistry than I had planned to cover, but there are plenty of interesting things that you can take away from that list:

1) The number of different phytochemicals found in plants is VAST: I do not exaggerate when I say that there are tens of thousands that we know about and possibly millions yet to be identified and analyzed as to their precise molecular structures.

2) Many of these phytochemicals like curcumin are unstable and thus defy clinical analysis because we do not know which form is the effective one.

3) Although we have come a long way in our ability to analyze the molecular structures of organic compounds, many still defy this analysis and remain a mystery as to their actual molecular construction.

4) Many primary essential nutrients to the human body including Vitamins A and E are not isolated molecular forms but members of classes of phytochemicals that contain hundreds of similar compounds that may be significant to human nutrition as well.

So all of those molecules are out there in all of the natural whole foods and we have NO IDEA which ones are of great value not just as simple nutrients but as potential and powerful remedials that can help prevent various diseases and ailments or even help us to resist and recover from the effects of those maladies after they appear. And even if we could analyze the molecular structure of every phytochemical in every single plant on Earth, clinical trials take time, and it would take eons to test them all. And to make matters worse, the scientists always want to isolate a single chemical in order to test it and quite often they LOSE their effectiveness when all of the rest of the chemicals in the natural food they were isolated from are missing.

END OF CHAPTER QUIZ

1. Resveratrol is:
   A. A phenolic compound (contains benzene rings)
   B. A powerful antioxidant
   C. Found in significant quantities in grapes, raisins, etc.
   D. All of the above.
   Answer: D. Resveratrol, found in grapes, is a powerful antioxidant and a stilbenoid, a subcategory of the phenolic phytonutrients.

2. Which two vitamins are rather simple terpenoids?
   A. Vitamin A and C
   B. Vitamin D and E
   C. Vitamin B1 and K
   D. Vitamin A and E
   Answer: D. Vitamin A is a simple diterpene and Vitamin E is a terpenol better known as a phytosterol.

According to the information from the previous list these can be categorized as the tetraterpenoids (a.k.a. carotenes and xanthophylls) triterpenoids, diterpenoids, monoterpenoids and the phytosterols. With 1,100 identified tetraterpenoids and over 200 plant sterols already known, there are very likely well over 2,000 terpenoids (that we have identified) and they are found in all plants and many animals produce these simple hydrocarbons as well.

THE TETRATERPENOIDS

These are all based on the basic molecular structure consisting of 40 carbon atoms and are the largest molecules of the terpenoid category of compounds. There are plenty of very important tetra-terpenoids including many that are essential nutrients to humans.

THE CAROTENES and BETA-CAROTENE

The carotenes are very common in edible raw plant foods including beta-carotene which imparts the characteristic orange color to the most commonly seen variety of carrots (they have been hybridized and can every color of the rainbow) and it is a water-soluble (safe to overindulge) powerful antioxidant precursor to Vitamin A and the body can break the beta-carotene molecule and turn it into Vitamin A with ease as needed. Vitamin A is not just responsible for maintaining eye health but it is also required by the skin and it should come as no surprise that excesses of beta-carotene are transported to the skin for storage until needed. But that's not all, beta-carotene is a powerful antioxidant and has been shown to prevent and combat many forms of cancer as well as many forms of heart disease.[1]

LYCOPENE

This is also a carotene and while it is found in carrots mainly because it is a precursor to beta-carotene, it is found in much higher quantities in other commonly found foods. Lycopene is one of the most powerful antioxidants known and there has been plenty of clinical research done on it. The health benefits of lycopene sound almost too good to be true, but researchers have shown that lycopene:

1) Is a powerful anti-inflammatory and may help ease arthritis.
2) Helps prevent and combat several forms of cancer including breast cancer, prostate cancer, and others.
3) Prevents and fights cataracts and blocks many actions in the cells of the eye that lead to Macular Degeneration.
4) Alleviates neuropathic pain caused by nerve damage in the soft tissues or other difficult to combat forms of neurological pain like phantom limb pain of amputees.
5) Prevents and even corrects many forms of neurological damage including but not limited to the damage caused

by MSG (monosodium glutamate,) seizures, Alzheimer's Disease, etc.

6) Linked to the prevention and correction of many heart diseases including coronary heart disease, myocardial ischemia, atherosclerosis, etc.

7) Helps reduce oxidative stress in the bones (its power as an antioxidant shines here) which can help keep the bones from becoming weak and brittle.[2]

If that's not enough to convince you that you need lycopene in your diet I don't know anything with more health benefits and a better VERIFIED track record from direct clinical trials.

THE XANTHOPHYLLS

These are found in all green plants and impart a yellow color to the leaves of some plants like variegated ginger, but xanthophylls are found in all green plant leaves and it does do some photosynthesis as well hence the name. Xanthophylls are not nearly as efficient as chlorophyll but are much more easily produced. It is sort of like the plant has a few very high priced free agents (the chlorophylls) and a bunch of lower priced veterans and rookies to round out the team. Some plants like spinach in particular do invest a lot of resources in making a lot more chlorophyll than xanthophylls, but they still have a lot of both. Two xanthophylls that have come under scrutiny of late are Zeaxanthin and Lutein.[3]

ZEAXANTHIN and LUTEIN

These two tetraterpenoids are xanthophylls, yellow photosynthesis molecules found in many plants in trace amounts. There has been a lot of hype about them recently concerning eye health and while most researchers indicate that most tests have been inconclusive, there are some undeniable facts about these two phytonutrients:

1) Both are found in heavy concentrations in the eye and therefore MUST play a significant role in human vision.

2) They are both very powerful antioxidants which means that they too will protect the eye just like lycopene.

Most of the trouble with these two as well as lycopene is the fact that they seem to lose their effectiveness when taken as isolated supplements. Fortunately, there are many superfoods loaded with them and in their natural whole food forms they truly shine. In fact many studies with lycopene were conducted by treating the test group of patients with natural foods and NOT supplements. Zeaxanthin and Lutein on the other hand were tested with supplements.[4]

THE TRITERPENES

These are smaller molecules consisting of 30 carbon atoms and their attendant hydrogen atoms with a few additional attached groups that distinguish them from one another. One major group found in many plants are the SAPONINS.[5]

ASTAXANTHIN

This newcomer to the research arena has shown some

incredible properties: 1) It is one of the most powerful antioxidants known to science, 2) It has all of the amazing powers of the other carotenes including protecting and improving heart health, 3) improves cognitive brain function, 4) helps prevent and fight cancer, 5) It has shown strong anti-inflammatory properties, 6) rejuvenates and protects the skin and eyes, 7) Boosts metabolism, and 8) Boosts male fertility. None of this is surprising when researchers have reported that Astaxanthin is SIX THOUSAND TIMES more potent as an antioxidant than Vitamin C, 550 TIMES more potent than Vitamin E, and 40 TIMES more potent than beta-carotene which is one of the strongest and most powerful antioxidants you can find. While astaxanthin can be found in supplements, these can have negative side effects because the nutrient is SO POWERFUL. But many natural foods have it and you would be wise to include it in your regular natural whole foods diet.[6]

THE SAPONINS

This subgroup of triterpenes get their name from "Saponaria" the genus of the soapwort plant which was used since ancient times to make natural soap and the saponins do indeed create foam when mixed with water and shaken. Many are toxic in large amounts and it is believed that the plants use these compounds to deter herbivores. But they are extremely toxic to insects which are usually a far greater nuisance to plants (and the most likely targets of the saponins) than grazing animals and in small doses saponins in livestock feed reduce the breakdown of their waste into ammonia which is extremely toxic to the animals especially when large numbers of them are confined in small areas.

There is evidence that saponins help the digestive tract with the absorption of other nutrients and they also increase cellular membrane permeability (allow molecules to move into and out of the cells more easily.)

Many different saponin rich plants have been used by indigenous people to poison fish as a form of getting the fish easily. The saponins change the properties of water (like soap) and the fish literally drown because their gills can no longer absorb oxygen from the water. Small amounts of saponins in our foods are also non-toxic and thus the saponins can and do kill the fish while leaving them perfectly safe to eat. With that said I would not recommend chewing on soapwort roots any time soon and you would probably never have to or want to eat saponin rich plants, but these compounds may be beneficial in trace amounts.[7]

OLEANOLIC ACID

One of the many interesting phytonutrients found in olive oil, oleanolic acid has been shown to have hematoprotective powers (it helps protect red blood cells) and researchers report that this substance has antitumor and antiviral properties as well.[Z]

Researchers have also found that this amazing phytonutrient has shown promise in fighting HIV and similar diseases. Scientists are actually pursuing synthetic variants of this compound as possible treatments for HIV and other related viruses. So like I have often said, the ONLY salad dressing worth using is oil (olive oil to be specific) and vinegar.[8]

BETULINIC ACID

There are many more triterpenoid acids and they all have amazing potential but there has been little clinical trial research done on them. Betulinic acid however, has shown great promise in several studies where it has been found to possess antiretroviral (retards HIV and related viruses) properties like oleanolic acid, as well as antimalarial, and antitumor properties including action as a selective inhibitor of human melanoma; one of the worst, most aggressive and difficult to treat forms of cancer. Clearly the triterpenes include many possible future wonder drugs.[9]

THE DITERPENES

I have yet to find much research into this group of compounds which is not to say that it is devoid of beneficial phytonutrients and remedials. I am still in the process of researching phytonutrients in general and I am sure that some diterpenes will show up so stay tuned; I plan to write many future volumes in this series on the amazing powers of all-natural whole foods and their constituents.

Of course we have all heard of RETINOL a.k.a. VITAMIN A which is one of the first essential nutrients for the human body ever identified by science and it happens to be a diterpenoid and I am confident that there are many more diterpenes in our whole foods with amazing properties and benefits to human health.[10]

THE MONOTERPENES

These relatively small hydrocarbons pack a powerful punch and have a wide range of commercial uses from cleansers and antibacterials to flavorings for processed foods, drinks, and other products like mouthwash.[11]

PERILLYL ALCOHOL

This monoterpene has been used in everything from cosmetics to cleansers but in 2015 research began on perillyl alcohol (a precursor to limonene found in several natural whole foods) as a treatment for certain forms of brain cancer. Perillyl alcohol is definitely on the menu![12]

THE PHYTOSTEROLS

This is the last subgroup of the terpenoids but far from the least in terms of numbers of compounds and their potential benefits to human health. One of the most powerful and indeed ESSENTIAL phytonutrients for humans is a phytosterol known as alpha-tocopherol or by its common name: VITAMIN E.[13]

BETA-SITOSTEROL

Beta-sitosterol has been produced as a supplement intended to lower cholesterol for years although most experts argue that there has been no conclusive study showing that it does. This does not mean that it is ineffective however. This compound is found in many foods and I will point out the best sources in an upcoming chapter.[14]

END OF CHAPTER QUIZ

1. One of the most powerful antioxidants known to science is:
    A. Vitamin C
    B. Vitamin E
    C. Beta-carotene
    D. Astaxanthin
    Answer: D. Astaxanthin is 6,000 TIMES more potent than Vitamin C, 550 TIMES more potent than Vitamin E, and 40 times more potent than beta-carotene.
2. Another amazingly powerful tetraterpenoid antioxidant is:
    A. Lycopene
    B. Zeaxanthin
    C. Lutein
    D. All of the above
    Answer: D. All three of these tetraterpenoids have been found to have potent antioxidant powers although lycopene is the only one proven conclusively to be an effective nutrient.
3. Several triterpenes have shown amazing preventative and curative powers as:
    A. Antivirals
    B. Antioxidants
    C. Anti-aging treatments
    D. None of the above
    Answer: A. Oleanolic acid and Betulinic acid have shown significant efficacy and promise as antivirals against HIV and other related viruses which have proven to be enormously resistant to most other antiviral treatments.
4. The most famous diterpenoid (also an essential nutrient) is:
    A. Vitamin A
    B. Vitamin C
    C. Lycopene
    D. Vitamin E
    Answer: Vitamin A or retinol is the most well known diterpene.
5. The most famous (and also essential nutrient) phytosterol is:
    A. Vitamin A
    B. Vitamin C
    C. Lycopene
    D. Vitamin E
    Answer: Vitamin E is the most well known phytosterol.

We covered quite a bit of ground in the preceding chapter and it is important to understand that we are only dotting through the thousands of known, and potentially millions of unknown as yet, phytonutrients. And the phenolics are a HUGE group of compounds and there are a LOT of significant ones in terms of human nutrition and that also play roles as curatives and preventatives for just about every system in the human body.

THE MONOPHENOLS

If you remember the discussions in the previous chapter that introduced the major classes of phytochemicals then you know that "phenol" or "phenyl" refers to that symmetrical ring of six bonded carbon atoms. So the monophenols are generally rather small molecules that contain just one of these rings. Though simple, they have some serious punch.[15]

CARVACROL and CARNOSOL

Both of these are found in many herbs and spices and they lend some of the pungent aromas and strong flavors to them as well. Both are being researched and have shown efficacy as antibacterials and as antioxidants they have shown promise in targeting and killing cancerous cells. There is no question that you should start using that battery of spices that have been collecting dust in your kitchen cabinet![16]

THE FLAVONOIDS and ISOFLAVONOIDS

This is the first major subdivision of the polyphenols which comprise the bulk of the phenols and are simply all phenols that have more than one benzyl ring of six carbon atoms within the molecular structure. There are over 5,000 identified flavonoids so far and we have very likely only just scratched the surface of them. They are found in virtually all plants edible or not and are primarily used by the plants for color in stems and leaves, but mostly for flowers and fruits. Although they provide color to the reproductive systems of the plants, which is important for attracting pollinators like bees, as well as animals to come and take the fruits (which helps disperse the seeds) they also play many other roles in the plants as well and have become an enormous factor in human nutrition too.[17]

MYRICETIN – A FLAVONOL

This flavonoid is found in many plants and has the unusual property of being able to act both as an antioxidant as well as an oxidant. Studies of myricetin have shown that it has antimutagenic properties; a fancy way of saying that it proactively prevents cancer by protecting the DNA in cells from being mutated. Antimutagens are few and far between and they are the first line of defense against all forms of cancer. All of the B vitamins and Vitamin E have this amazing power which is why I so strongly urge everyone to get at least the 100% RDA of them all especially from natural whole foods. And it certainly cannot hurt to load up on as many additional antimutagens as we can find to bolster our defenses against one of the worst modern epidemic scourges: cancer.

But myricetin does even more: as an oxidant it has shown antiviral potential, as an antioxidant it has shown potential to retard thrombosis (build up and unnecessary activation of blood platelets causing dangerous internal blood clots,) myricetin has shown promise as having the ability to prevent insulin resistance by directly participating in blood sugar transport biochemistry (may prevent diabetes and is currently being researched as a treatment for diabetes,) potential power to prevent atherosclerosis and other forms of heart disease, potential for reducing oxidative stress in brain cells (prevent neuronal damage and degradation which lead to such ailments as Alzheimer's disease and Parkinson's disease,) and finally, myricetin has been shown to interfere directly with inflammatory pathways meaning that it has the potential to be one of the most powerful anti-inflammatory nutrients known to man. And this is JUST ONE of the thousands of flavonoids and most have yet to be investigated.[18]

HESPERIDIN – A FLAVANONE

Research has only just begun on this flavonoid found in citrus fruits with the highest concentration found in the peels. Citrus have a unique classification of fruit form – made of sections, each made out of bundles of juice filled sacks called a "hesperidium" – from which this compound's name was taken. It is too early for researchers to confirm its power as an anticancer nutrient, but if it is suspected, then there is likely a reason for that suspicion and since citrus are the very best sources of so many other nutrients, it is nice to have this one coming along for the ride as well.[19]

APIGENIN – A FLAVONE

Although this one has only been tested in test tubes and mice (the very early stages of research) the outlook is promising. It might be able to stimulate the growth of new brain cells, and has shown positive action in the interference of the destructive pathways of brain cell degradation caused by Alzheimer's disease in vitro (means in the test tube, not in live animals or humans which is called "in vivo") and it has shown the ability to reduce the resistance of cancer stem cells (that are the primary targets of importance in fighting certain malignant cancers that are difficult to treat) as well as the ability to stimulate the repair of the kidneys caused by destructive chemicals given to mice.

The research is in the early phases, but it does sound like apigenin could assist in the recovery from brain injuries caused by a host of maladies ranging from stroke to Alzheimer's disease as well as help chemotherapy have a greater effect on targeted cancer cells making the treatments faster and more effective and if it can induce repair in the kidneys, that alone would make it a true wonder drug since kidney tonics are some of the rarest natural remedies known. In other words, once your kidneys fail, they don't get better and the person is doomed to a life of regular trips to the hospital for dialysis.[20]

THE CATECHINS – FLAVAN-3-OLS

There has been a lot of study on this group of compounds found in many foods since the 1930's. It has been established in studies back then as well as more recent studies conducted in Europe that catechins do improve capillary permeability and lower blood pressure especially in those that have very high systolic pressure (the lower number that indicates the pressure between the heart beats.) The trouble with the catechins is that they are numerous and often found in bunches in natural foods and our bodies are definitely on the lookout for them and they are very quickly and readily absorbed and sent to the liver where it transforms them quickly into a series of "metabolites" or modified forms which are then sent on into the bloodstream for use by the rest of the body.

To researchers this is a problem because the catechins in their naturally occurring forms are not the nutrients that have the positive effects in our bodies; it is the metabolites that the liver builds out of them that are the keys. We however, are not interested in patenting things to make billions, we are interested in good health and the catechins are definitely on the menu.[21]

THE ANTHOCYANIDINS

This is another large group with many members although only one or two are usually present in any specific food source. Although they are named for the color blue ("cyan" in the name) they can actually produce a whole host of colors in plants from predominantly dark purple (eggplant) to medium blue (blueberries) to even red (strawberries.) I am well aware of the recent concern about many of these thin skinned berries and other foods being trouble because they can absorb pesticides and fungicides into them through those thin skins, so even washing them will not protect you from being poisoned by those chemicals. And there is no denying the fact that if you eat whole natural plant foods purchased in the produce section of your local grocery store, they are ALL bathed in these chemicals. Even many so-called "Organic" foods can be laced with these poisons because the FDA has a very low set of standards on what can carry that "Organic" label; all a subject for an upcoming volume in this series.

In the meantime, the anthocyanidins are currently being studied but they have shown that they have many health benefits including: prevention or reduction of high blood pressure as well as reduced risk of myocardial infarction and heart attack, improved immune system, prevention of cancer, improved cognitive function, improved metabolism, and improved vision and eye health. Of course this sounds a lot like the benefits of antioxidants in general and that's because they are antioxidants.

Many different foods are loaded with anthocyanidins and anthocyanins (very closely related group, so you don't necessarily have to eat blueberries laced with chemicals (even though they are one of the densest sources and most well studied members of this group of nutrients and have shown most of the remarkable health benefits listed above.)[22]

THE PHYTOESTROGENS

Although related closely to estrogen found in all mammals and believed to be a plant defense against grazing animals by reducing their fertility rates, this is believed to be very effective on ruminant digestive tracts, but not humans who have a significantly different digestive system. Some researchers believe that the phyto-estrogens may help prevent or fight breast cancer and other maladies of the female reproductive system, but caution that results so far have been rather inconclusive. Again we must remember that many such studies involve extracts of the pure compound and NOT the natural whole foods which can and does affect the efficacy of many of these complex molecules. One study has shown that Secoisolariciresinol (I am not going to even attempt to pronounce that one!) has shown positive results in reducing the risk of cardiovascular disease.[23]

SILYMARIN – A FLAVONOLIGNAN

This and a host of other similar compounds, all precursors and metabolites found in milk thistle have been shown to promote liver health by helping the liver purge toxins that it accumulates as part of its job of filtering them out of the foods we eat and also by promoting new cell growth. While silymarin itself is suspected as being the "active ingredient," because the plant contains a whole host of related compounds I suspect that it is this whole group that will have the best results. Most supplements do in fact contain whole, dried, powdered leaves which is excellent.[24]

RESVERATROL – A STILBENOID

While resveratrol has received a lot of attention in the past decade, most researchers insist that there is little if any evidence that it has a positive effect on human health. However, numerous studies have shown the positive effects of grapes, grape juice, raisins and even wine on human health. This is a clear case in which using the purified compound LOWERS THE EFFECTIVENESS of the constituent. The one thing we do know is that resveratrol is an antioxidant and that grapes and their natural by-products do improve the cardiovascular system. Personally, I wouldn't pay for refined resveratrol supplements (or refined supplements of any kind for that matter) but I do drink at least 2 whole cups of Pure Concord grape juice per day. And there have been times in my life in which that was the only thing I took up again while trying to get back to my whole natural food diet, and I could FEEL the difference it makes. So, I don't care if it is the resveratrol or something else, or the combination of everything in it that makes it work; I only care that it does work.[25]

CURCUMIN

This one is HUGE in terms of the attention it has received of late and the fact that the scientists and profiteers are all saying that it doesn't work. Of course this is due primarily to the fact that the scientists cannot prove which isomer is the effective one and the molecule does change based solely on the conditions around it and there is no way to get inside the human cells and determine which form it is in when it does its work for us. This means that it cannot be synthesized or patented for use because the actual pathway that the molecule works on cannot be determined.

So the scientists can't prove anything and the profiteers cannot make their billions off of it, but that does not change the fact that it could indeed be very effective and there is plenty of anecdotal evidence that it does work. Whether curcumin is an actual antimutagen (prevents damage to DNA,) or an antitumor agent ((specifically targets and kills cancerous cells) may never be determined or fully understood because the molecule is inherently unstable, but many people including medical doctors worldwide are convinced that curcumin can and does have noticeable anticancer properties and may be one of nature's most potent nutrients for humans to combat this dreaded category of diseases.[26]

TANNINS

This is a huge family of molecules that are themselves physically very large molecules and the tannins are found throughout all plants from edible berries to trees. A species of mangrove found in large numbers in Florida release large quantities of tannins into the standing water where they grow turning it brown (this effect is also produced by tannins leeching out of the dead leaves and wood in many wetland forests.) There are in fact many rivers in Florida that flow with this brownish water that I affectionately call "tea rivers" because it is the tannins in tea that turn the drink brown.

Traditionally, tannins have always been considered either neutral or worse; antinutritional. However, new research indicates that tannins may indeed have a positive effect, but it is still too early to tell. Overindulgence in tannin rich foods like brown tea has been shown to cause renal problems, but overindulgence in this drink is likely due to caffeine addiction and any such addiction can lead to heavy overindulgence which can always lead to serious physiological problems.[27]

THE PHENOLIC ACIDS

There are plenty of these including salicylic acid, a.k.a. aspirin as well as vanillic acid, gallic acid, ellagic acid and tannic acid (tannins that acquire the –O-O-H group and become organic acids.) We all know the potential benefit of aspirin although in its purified form, it tends to knock holes in people's stomachs. We have not pursued most of the others that play key roles in the actual flavors of the foods that contain them, but that does not mean that they have no other effect (positive or negative) on the human body.[28]

THE HYDROXYCINNAMIC ACIDS

These include cinnamic acid, ferulic acid and coumarin (the distinct aroma of a freshly mowed lawn) to name just a few. They are found in many different foods and contribute to their various flavors in conjunction with many other organic acids and flavonoids. It is the actual combinations of all of these constituents and their relative quantities that impart the flavors on all of the natural plant foods that we eat. Ferulic acid is found in many foods and to date almost no research has been conducted as to its potential health benefits although one study did show promise in its use in conjunction with Vitamins C and E in improving skin health.[29]

CAPSAICIN

Are there health benefits from eating red hot chili peppers? There are actually reports that it can have positive effects ranging from helping people lose weight, to improving cardiovascular health and capsaicin (it is actually a group of similar compounds produced by many different plants) has been used as a topical pain reliever for arthritis. It works in this way because it literally overloads the nerves pain receptors and effectively numbs them for a time. Personally, I would never recommend rubbing jalapenos on your skin, but I do love them in my chili and home made salsa![30]

GINGEROL

One of the main constituents of ginger root that gives it its distinctive spicy flavor, gingerol has been shown in limited preliminary investigations to have a positive effect on rheumatoid arthritis as well as targeting cancerous cells preferentially and killing them. The anecdotal and folklore claims of ginger's healing powers range from being effective at helping overcome everything from the common cold, to prevention and treatment of just about every other disease. One thing is for sure, gingerol is potent and research into its healing powers has only just begun.[31]

THE GLUCOSINOLATES

This is another major category of phytonutrients that all contain at least one sulfur atom. There are many major subcategories and research has only just begun into the critical roles they play in human nutrition.[32]

THE INDOLES

This is a major subcategory of the sulfur compounds found in all plants including IAA (Indole Acid Amine) which is a root growth stimulation hormone produced by all plants. Indoles are indeed found in all plants and play a vast number of roles in their biochemistry and many indoles are well known narcotics. But not all indoles are "bad" and many are being researched for their positive effects on human health.

INDOLE-3-CARBINOL

This constituent of many vegetables is currently being investigated for its known antioxidant powers that include suspected anti-carcinogenic properties as well as the ability to prevent and treat many forms of heart disease.[34]

THE BETALAINS

Another major category of the phenolics, betalains are found in great abundance in beets and a few other edible plants. Although a relatively small group of compounds and investigation has only just begun, a few have shown great promise.[35]

INDICAXANTHIN

A betalain, indicaxanthin is a very powerful antioxidant that has shown greater efficacy in the treatment of at least one disease over treatments based on either Vitamin C or Vitamin E. This alone should be an indication that the betalains, which beets are loaded with, are of great potential importance as a health promoting nutrient. So be sure to eat your beets![36]

THE CHLOROPHYLLS

This is actually a relatively small group and we all know that plants use chlorophyll for photosynthesis. But its presence in virtually all plant foods, particularly the leaves like lettuce and spinach and their relatives means that mankind evolved eating chlorophyll rich foods and it is no surprise that we absorb it and we use it, although our bodies do deconstruct the molecule primarily to get at that magnesium atom which we use in countless enzymes found in virtually all cells in the human body.

Chlorophylls have also been shown to be powerful detoxifiers for the liver as well. So eat your leafy greens![37]

THE OTHER ORGANIC ACIDS

This is a huge grab bag of phytonutrients that basically do not fall into any of the other major categories of molecules and they are found in virtually all plants and include: phytic acid, oxalic acid, tartaric acid, anacardic acid, and malic acid to name just a few. While these all play roles in shaping the flavors of the foods they are found in, we have seen that many plant nutrients start out as simple pigments like the flavonoids, and then turn out to be major influences on the flavors of the foods (hence the name of the group) and also turn out to be very important for human health because many of them are for example, antioxidants. But it is also important to remember that a phytonutrient does not have to be an antioxidant in order to be a very potent nutrient or remedial.

END OF CHAPTER QUIZ

1. What two monophenols are found in some spices?

A. Carvacrol and carnosol
B. Myricetin and hesperidin
C. Silymarin and resveratrol
D. None of the above are found in spices
Answer: D. Carnosol and carvocrol lend their warm pungent aromas to several spices and are suspected of being very healthy for the human body in small amounts.

2. Which of the following has the unusual property of acting like both a powerful antioxidant as well as a powerful oxidant?
A. Resveratrol
B. Silymarin
C. Myricetin
D. No nutrient has this ability
Answer: D. Myricetin can act as both an antioxidant as well as an oxidant making it of particular interest to investigators.

3. Which known antioxidant has not been proven through clinical trials to show health benefits despite extensive research?
A. Resveratrol
B. Silymarin
C. Myricetin
D. Hesperidin
Answer: A. Resveratrol has been researched extensively and has shown no conclusive evidence that it can serve as a preventative or a curative to any ailments despite the fact that it is a known and powerful antioxidant. Myricetin and hesperidin research has only just begun and silymarin is difficult to test because milk thistle contains dozens of related molecules.

4. Which of the following kinds of phytonutrients lend a blue color to foods?
A. Flavonoids
B. Glucosinolates
C. Phenolic acids
D. Anthocyanodins
Answer: D. The anthocyanodins are common phytonutrients that make the foods blue like eggplant and blueberries.

4. Which of the following kinds of phytonutrients contain at least one sulfur atom?
A. Flavonoids
B. Glucosinolates
C. Phenolic acids
D. Anthocyanodins
Answer: A. The glucosinolates are all compounds that contain at least one sulfur atom and are often very biologically active compounds like the indoles.

AMINES and OTHER NITROGEN-BASED COMPOUNDS
This is an enormous group that includes the amino acids and therefore all plant proteins as well as most enzymes and other metabolic structures. The "ines" (pronounced "EENS") certainly do abound in plants and you have definitely heard about many of them including: CAFFEINE, NICOTINE, MORPHINE, and COCAINE, to name a few. We certainly do seem to like them a lot and this is because they have such powerful effects on the human physiology. We might say that this group includes some of the most BIOACTIVE phytochemicals known.[57]

THE NINE ESSENTIAL AMINO ACIDS
Although covered in Vol. 3 a quick recap is in order here. It is also important to note that while all nine are found in virtually all proteins including those in plants, methionine and lysine are in lower concentration in plants than in animal proteins. It is also important to remember that there are many more amino acids in all proteins than just these nine. The difference is that the FDA has issued an RDA (Recommended Daily Allowance) for these nine meaning that they must be present in your daily diet. The RDA for them stipulates 110g of protein (specifically "Complete Protein" that contains ample amounts of all nine – in other words ANIMAL protein of any kind) or about 4 ounces and should be considered a bare minimum requirement.[38]

1) **ISOLEUCINE** – This amino acid is critical to the formation of hemoglobin in the blood and also helps muscle growth in children in particular. KIDS NEED A LOT OF PROTEIN, adults need it too because most of our organ systems are constantly in the process of regeneration and renewal and therefore constantly engaged in cell division and growth. Amino acid (protein) deficient diets low in isoleucine lead to slow development and poor overall health as well as progressive degeneration of all bodily systems and premature aging notably in the skin and hair, but also reduced brain function and weakened and inflamed joints.

2) **HISTIDINE** – Foods high in histidine (again found in most protein rich foods) assist in detoxification of the body and proper brain function.

3) **LEUCINE** – Leucine has been shown to help regulate insulin and therefore normalize blood sugar levels. People who are eating a low protein diet or suffer from chronic leucine deficiency are at risk and this can play a contributing role in the development of diabetes or hypoglycemia. If you haven't noticed yet, BLOOD SUGAR and its proper function is one of the MOST COMPLEX metabolic functions in the human body and there is a VAST number of essential nutrients and other biochemical processes and organ systems at work to keep it running properly. This is indeed one system in our body that we LIVE or DIE on and it has a

LOT of moving parts. A healthy balanced natural whole foods diet is the very best way to make sure that none of those gears in that massive and complicated system gets fouled up.

4) **LYSINE** – Lysine has been shown to play a critical role in the body's proper usage of CALCIUM and supports proper bone health. All of the CONCRETE tablets (Calcium phosphate supplements) on Earth WILL NOT prevent osteoporosis without LYSINE (proper all natural whole foods diet rich in animal protein) although they should be able to give you a baseball sized kidney stone quickly enough.

5) **METHIONINE** – This is one of the amino acids that contains sulfur. You would expect to find it in the sulfurous foods like eggs and broccoli and you would be quite right. Methionine is critical to the construction and maintenance of cartilage in the body and why people on low protein diets get joint problems.

6) **PHENYLALANINE** – Try to say THAT three times fast. Phenylalanine (I remember it as "fennih-lala-neen") is critical to thyroid health and helps the gland produce its hormones, the ones built on those two weird minerals: iodine and selenium. Low protein diets consisting of mostly GARBAGE calories in packaged and processed foods can also reduce thyroid function and land you in a world of trouble with lower metabolism and obesity. Overweight people who also have a problem staying warm (often complain about the "freezing" temperature in an air-conditioned office) ARE SUFFERING FROM SEVERELY REDUCED METABOLIC RATE caused by DEPRESSED THYROID FUNCTION. You can piece everything together from these books but I will include an upcoming volume on this global epidemic problem and how you can EASILY FIX IT.

7) **TRYPTOPHAN** – Often thought of as the reason we get drowsy after eating a ton of turkey on Thanksgiving, that drowsiness is actually caused by the very high levels of LACTIC ACID in turkey meat. LACTIC ACID is what your body produces as a by-product of lengthy exercise and what makes your muscles ache and makes you feel exhausted. Tryptophan is an essential amino acid incorporated into every protein in every cell of your body and virtually all high protein foods have just as much as turkey, so let's get that TRUTH taken care of once and for all shall we: LACTIC ACID NOT TRYPTOPHAN. (Obviously I am tired of arguing about this with everyone. I don't know where that DISINFORMATION started, but it is time to put a stop to it already.) Tryptophan is involved in proper neurotransmitter and brain function. Ironically it makes you MORE ALERT and improves concentration, mood, etc. It has the OPPOSITE EFFECT of LACTIC ACID. I am done with my rant. Believe what you want.

8) **THREONINE** – This amino acid is also linked to proper central nervous system function as well as heart, liver and immune health.

A chronic low protein diet could land you in BIG TROUBLE if you are putting all of those systems at risk.

9) **VALINE** – Body-builders know what valine is for: proper muscle growth, strength and endurance. Even though we do not necessarily want to look like those guys (and gals!) we still need it for proper muscle formation and maintenance.[38]

COMPLETE PROTEIN

It is important to note that no plant has Complete Protein although some do have higher levels of methionine and lysine they are all deficient in these critical amino acids. This however, is only a problem for vegans because all forms of animal protein are by definition Complete Protein; in other words they all have ample concentrations of the nine essential amino acids.

BETAINE

This is another amino acid, but not considered one of the nine essential ones. It is made from choline and though it is named after the beet, it happens to have its highest concentrations in wheat. So westerners are certainly getting ample supplies of it in their diet and it has been shown to significantly lower homocysteine in the blood which helps reduce plaque build up and the risk of other heart diseases. For those who are gluten-intolerant, beets are the next best source of betaine.[39]

PROTEIN IN OUR DIET

Protein is the basic main construction material of all living cells from the simplest archaebacteria to the protozoans to all plants, animals, and fungi. Every living cell on Earth is essentially a protein sack filled with water and other protein structures. Even DNA is essentially a huge very special protein strand made out of four different amino acids. The series of these "base-pairs" along the DNA molecule is what carries the encoded information about every physical aspect of the specific species of creature that will grow from the fertilized ovum cell called a zygote. It should be obvious that children need lots of protein because they have a lot of growing to do and all of that growth involves the creation of massive numbers of new cells and those are all made out of proteins. But adults are continuously regenerating as well; cells continuously die and are continuously replaced in nearly every organ system in the body from the skin to the bones and everything in between.

And it is precisely because of this ongoing regeneration process that we must have ample quantities of protein, Complete Protein, in our daily diet. And while only these nine amino acids have been specified by the FDA as "essential" nutrients it is important to remember that they are a governmental agency just trying to do their best and they are certainly not a reflection of reality or specifically of nature and what our bodies actually do need.

So while we may easily make our own amino acids, other than these nine essential ones, what do you think our cells make the other amino acids out of? It is likely not air and water and a few nitrates (that's the amazing power of plants, by the way, through photosynthesis they CAN do that) it is much more likely that we need to load up on amines and other amino acids in order to have the raw materials for our cells to build other amino acids that they need. The bottom line is that we must eat protein to provide the raw materials that our bodies need in order to keep up with the continuous regeneration processes going on in all organ systems in the body throughout our entire lives and Complete Protein is the very best source of this basic and fundamental set of nutrients.

THE CARBOHYDRATES

While most of the phytonutrients in the preceding chapters could be called carbohydrates in the broadest sense, the term is used primarily to refer to a group of nutrients that have a specific structure and ratio of carbon to hydrogen to oxygen in them. The two major subcategories are monosaccharides or simple sugars including hexose found in wheat, pentose found in rye and oats, fructose found in most fruits, as well as glucose which our liver makes from all of the other sugars that we eat and sends that form into our bloodstream for all cells to use as metabolic fuel. The polysaccharides are an enormous group that includes the starches and most fats like the polyunsaturated fats which are found in most plants and refined into the various vegetable oil products like Canola oil, as well as many other substances like cellulose that are in essence fiber because we cannot digest them.

Since the carbohydrates are the direct source of metabolic energy that we use to actually function, and are measured in the form of calories, you could say that the carbohydrates form a large bulk percentage of most plant foods and are the number one phytonutrients that all humans need in order to function. If you do not get calories in your diet, then you emaciate and eventually starve to death.[58]

POLYUNSATURATED FATS

These are a significant group of carbohydrates found in many plant foods especially the seeds and nuts. While these are loaded with calories (more than an equal weight of sugars) they are also MUCH HEALTHIER forms of calories than refined sugar or animal fats.

OMEGA-6 FATTY ACIDS

These are getting a lot of attention and it is all negative. The problem is not the Omega-6's themselves, but rather the ratio of them in our diet versus the Omega-3's. A healthy ratio should be at least 3:1 Omega-3 to Omega-6 on a daily basis. Since the Omega-6's are in all vegetable oils (and almost all packaged and processed foods) while most people might not get ANY Omega-3 at all for days even weeks at a time, this is what is causing the health issues. The Omega-6's are good for you, but you must make sure that you are also getting plenty of the Omega-3's to compensate.[40]

OMEGA-3 FATTY ACID alpha-LINOLEIC ACID

These are also getting a lot of attention and it is all good. Aside from the hype, these compounds are tremendously good for you and contribute to prevention and even correction of heart disease, atherosclerosis, high cholesterol as well as improved liver health and brain function. The ONLY Omega-3 found in plants in alpha-Linoleic acid or ALA and it is relatively rare in most plant foods and is almost only found in certain seeds and nuts.[41]

* * *

Aside from oxygen and water, carbohydrates are actually ranked number three in terms of the amount by weight of the nutrients that our bodies need on a daily basis. The current established standard requirement for adults is approximately 2,000 calories per day. To put this into perspective, one of the most carbohydrate dense foods on Earth is honey. One tablespoon weighs about 21g and 17 grams of that is in the form of complex sugars which are pure carbohydrates that translate into about 60 calories (we are actually measuring the amount of energy they provide the human body and the unit is actually kilocalories but the "kilo" has simply been dropped making the word easier to say, I guess.) Since the average human needs about 2,000 calories per day and these 17 grams of honey provide 60 calories, then we would need 33.3 tablespoons of honey per day (and nothing else of course) which adds up to about 566 grams or 20 ounces. In the form of pure honey, a person would have to eat 1 ¼ POUNDS of honey each day to get 2,000 calories.

Luckily there are much denser forms of carbohydrates than sugars; that's the starches (long chains of sugars attached together that our digestive tracts can break down into the simple sugars out of which they are made) and the fats. The fats are large polymers (chains of repeating subunits like the starches) but are missing most of the oxygen atoms in each subunit which the sugars have. This makes the fats the densest most concentrated form of carbohydrate fuel and this is exactly why most plants, animals and people store their energy reserves in the form of fat.

While the simpler sugars have a density of about 100 calories per ounce, a glance at the nutrition label of my Canola oil reveals that 1 tablespoon weighs about 14 grams and contains 14 grams of fat (polyunsaturated fat, the GOOD kind) so it has been purified by the manufacturer and has only traces of other plant constituents left in it and that serving size is said to hold 120 calories. That's about 243 calories per ounce and only a little over half a pound would be needed to provide those 2,000 calories. Obviously I am not going to chug down half a pound of Canola oil. Aside from making me gag, the whole point here is to illustrate that even when the calorie content of the carbohydrate is concentrated, we still need a physically large amount of the food to get enough calories in our daily diet. And that proves the statement that after air and water, carbohydrates are the third largest nutrient by weight required by the human body on a daily basis and proteins totaling about 4 ounces per day are number four.

Incidentally, the only carbohydrates with a higher caloric density than the polyunsaturated fats found in plants are the saturated fats found in animal fats (including our own!)

END OF CHAPTER QUIZ

1. Complete Protein:
A. Contains all nine essential amino acids in sufficient quantities to satisfy our daily requirements
B. Contain many other amino acids that we can make ourselves, but it is good that we get them too
C. Is only found in animal foods.
D. All of the above
Answer: D. Animal foods are the only source of true Complete Protein that contains all nine essential amino acids in sufficient quantities to satisfy our daily requirements of them.

2. The average adult needs to consume about how much Complete Protein daily?
A. ¼ pound
B. A little over half a pound,
C. 1.25 pounds
D. All of the above are excessive
Answer: D. The average adult needs to consume at least a ¼ pound of Complete (animal) Protein daily for optimal health. Growing children and adults healing from injuries need even more.

3. Which of the following kinds of phytonutrients have the largest dietary daily intake requirements?
A. Terpenoids
B. Fiber
C. Proteins
D. Carbohydrates
Answer: D. We need more carbohydrates by weight in our daily intake than any other form of nutrient other than air and water.

4. The densest form of carbohydrates in terms of calories per ounce is:
A. Sugars
B. Starches
C. Polyunsaturated fats (vegetable oils)
D. Saturated fats (animal fats)
Answer: D. Saturated fats have the most calories per ounce.

Although the discussion has covered a lot of ground, it is now possible to come up with a "grand scheme" of things when discussing plant foods in particular.

COMPONENTS OF A TYPICAL PLANT FOOD

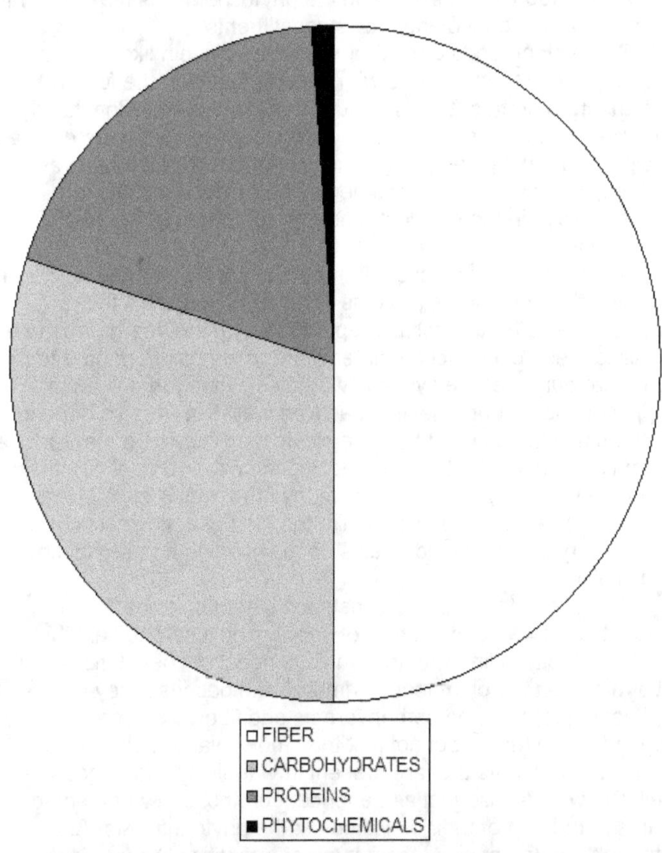

Every plant food you eat has this basic set of constituents: FIBER – those things we cannot digest, CARBOHYDRATES – sugars, starches, and polyunsaturated fats, PROTEIN – amino acids, and finally the PHYTOCHEMICALS – terpenoids, phenolics, glucosinolates, betalaines, chlorophylls, uncategorized organic acids, and the amines and other trace biologically active nitrogen compounds. The only major difference between one food, say oats, and another, say a banana, will be the actual sizes of these four major pie slices (the percentages of fiber, carbohydrates, proteins, and the remaining phytochemicals) in the specific food.

The significant small scale differences between two different plant foods will be the specific phytochemicals that each one brings as well as the specific molecular structures of their fiber, carbohydrates, and proteins. But you can be sure of one thing: they all have these four major components and the fiber, carbohydrates and proteins make up the vast majority of the mass of the plant food in question, and the phytochemicals make up only a very small minority of the food's constituents.

Some plant foods are extremely rich in protein like nuts and seeds which are also loaded with carbohydrates in the form of polyunsaturated fats (think peanut oil.) Others are predominantly fiber like celery (mostly fiber and water; it even takes more calories to digest it than it gives back in the way of absorbable carbs and protein.) But the "other" constituents, the phytochemicals, are almost always in the smallest amounts compared to the rest of the plant mass.

And there is no question that the components of any food that we need the most of are proteins and carbohydrates – the raw building blocks for our cells to reproduce, and the energy for them to utilize these construction materials. And we have adapted to the point that our digestive systems work best when there is an ample supply of fiber in our digestive tracts as well. But we also depend on the small minority of phytochemicals too. They hold many of the essential nutrients that our bodies depend on for proper health including vitamins, minerals, and many other major constituents that contribute to human health like the host of antioxidants and their sundry and profound effects on maintaining human health and vitality.

The percentages of the constituents happen to be in the amounts that we need in order of priority and it can be said that this is perfectly in line with the whole concept of coevolution: man was raised on the plant foods primarily and because they are highest in proteins and carbohydrates and fiber, we became dependent on these, but not just their molecular structures, but also in the amounts that are present in virtually all plant foods as well. But we are also just as dependent on those few percentage points of the rest of their constituents; the phytonutrients. And although we do not need them in great quantities like we do the carbohydrates, proteins and fiber, we do still need them in order to survive and more importantly to THRIVE.

This is exactly the central point of my argument that people should return to eating a diet primarily consisting of whole natural foods dominated by plant foods instead of eating predominantly prepackaged, prepared, precooked ("ready-to-eat") and processed foods. One of the primary culprits of these very low quality very low nutritional value types of foods is processed white wheat flour which has literally been processed down to the point where it is little more than wrecked wheat protein (gluten) and all of the amazing assortment of carbohydrates, and phytonutrients are GONE. Its cheap to make by the train load and it makes up the vast majority of the mass of most of these boxed and bagged "food" products that have basically the same nutritional value as giant pills of sawdust laced with flavors (mostly artificial) bright attractive colors (also mostly artificial) and tons of trash calories like processed sugar which is as dreadful for your health as it is addictive. And there are no phytonutrients in them so there are no antioxidants, no vitamins, no minerals or other essential nutrients unless they process, or worse synthesize them, and then throw them back in (like they do with many breakfast cereals.)

Rather than have a box full of sawdust laced with artificial flavors, colors and preservatives none of which do anything for you other than cause cancer, with a handful of essential nutrients cooked up in a laboratory rather than in their naturally occurring forms, I would prefer to eat foods with not only far superior levels of natural fiber, carbohydrates and proteins, but that are also loaded up with the phytonutrients as they occur in nature, the molecular forms that mankind was raised on from his humble beginnings; the foods that were good enough to transform monkeys into men.

In the preceding chapter I tracked down the actual amounts of the basic nutrient types that are needed by the average adult. It is important to realize that children and expecting and nursing mothers have far different nutritional requirements and parents and expecting or nursing mothers should definitely consult their doctors about the proper amounts of nutrients that they need. To recap our basic daily essential nutritional requirements:

1. **WATER** – While I have seen plenty of wildly differing estimates, inactive people should drink no less than a quart a day and double that is preferable. For active adults the amount should be a minimum of ½ gallon and double that is likely the best. Incidentally, most plants are about 85% to 90% water.

2. **CARBOHYDRATES** – In the form of simple sugars which provide about 100 calories per ounce you would need 20 ounces per day, or about 1 ¼ POUNDS of the stuff. Starches and polyunsaturated fats provide at least 240 calories per ounce reducing the average person's requirement for carbohydrate calories in these forms down to about ½ pound throughout the course of the day. Saturated animal fats are even higher and we do get some calories from proteins as well.

3. **PROTEINS** – The average adult requires at the very least about 4 ounces of Complete (animal) Protein in order to get sufficient quantities of the nine essential amino acids plus all of the others.

4. **FIBER** – Even though we technically do not digest this portion of the plant it is nonetheless a critical component of plant foods that our digestive tracts depend on and it also serves to absorb cholesterol in animal fats and prevent its absorption and plant cell

walls are reinforced with calcium compounds (which is what makes even green stemmed herbaceous plant's stems and leaves stiff) and our bodies can extract most of this trace mineral from these tissues even though they are mostly fiber.

5. **THE REST OF THE NUTRIENTS** – In plants this includes the phytochemicals, but the vast majority of them have yet to be identified much less tested in clinical trials. But we do know that we need Vitamin C and we only get it from plant foods. Therefore it is imperative to stick to whole natural foods as much as possible and to stop wasting time, money, and the stomach space by filling up on nonsense processed and packaged foods which are mostly devoid of any and all nutritional value and loaded up with trash calories which irritate the liver and manufactured chemicals that cause cancer.

END OF CHAPTER QUIZ

1. By far the nutrient we need the most of by weight per day is:
   A. Potassium
   B. Water
   C. Carbohydrates
   D. Proteins
   Answer: B. Water. A ½ gallon weighs about 4.85 pounds

2. By far the mineral we need the most of daily by weight is:
   A. Potassium
   B. Water
   C. Carbohydrates
   D. Proteins
   Answer: A. Potassium. Although not mentioned in this chapter, it is important enough to remember it. We need 3.2 grams per day which is enormous and most people do not get nearly that amount. It plays a critical role in nerve to muscle communication and without it the nerves cannot properly control the muscles including your HEART. It also plays a critical role in maintaining proper blood pressure and I suspect that the number one cause of high blood pressure and heart attacks in the U.S. is chronic severe potassium deficiency.

3. The largest nutrient by weight needed on a daily basis other than air and water is:
   A. Potassium
   B. Water
   C. Carbohydrates
   D. Proteins
   Answer: C. Carbohydrates. Without energy to burn, everything will shut down starting with your brain which needs a constant supply of glucose, a simple sugar prepared and delivered into the blood by the liver.

I included most of this material in chapter 1 of Vol.1 and 2, but it is important information and I have expanded it here.

STOP EATING POISON

If you really want to be healthy, that is, if you are looking for the most effective vitamin/mineral/supplement, then you are interested in being healthy and staying healthy. And rule number one in working toward being healthy is to stop eating poison and to start eating foods that do not have a significant percentage of poison in their ingredients.

Now I cannot possibly list for you all of the poisons that the greedy moneygrubbers are putting into our foods – that would require far too much paper and make the book rather expensive, but I can give you a few examples and I think you'll get the idea and be able to identify poisons in your food with no trouble after that.

Your stomach has one main function: to bathe everything that lands in it in a roughly pH 1 solution of Hydrochloric acid. This happens to be an incredibly dangerous and corrosive solution that while not as bad as alien blood (from the movie "Alien") it is one of the strongest acid solutions anywhere rivaling even the content of a car battery!

Anyway, the objective is to let that acid reduce complex molecules in the food into simpler ones and we're talking mainly about fats, starches and proteins all of which get cut down into smaller chunks, so starches are turned into sugars, proteins into amino acids and so on.

What is interesting about our stomach solution is that many things can dissolve in it, and if they dissolve in the solution, then it is also likely that they can be absorbed easily, either through the stomach lining itself which while unlikely is possible, but definitely through the intestinal walls and with great ease if the substance has been dissolved in the liquid released by the stomach into the beginning of the intestines called the duodenum. This section of intestine is tougher than the rest and can reabsorb the Hydrochloric acid that is still in the liquid called chyme (kyme) and get it out of there so it won't burn up the rest of your intestines.

Most, not all – we bear that in mind – Sodium salts will easily dissolve in the stomach acid. This frees the opposite piece in solution to be absorbed. For example, table salt is Sodium Chloride and it dissolves easily in the stomach solution yielding free Sodium ions and free Chloride ions. Both can be easily absorbed in the intestines thereafter. The Chloride ion is simply a Chlorine atom and you may have guessed from the nature of Hydrochloric acid, and the Mustard Gas used to kill thousands in World War 1 and the fact that adding it to your pool keeps microorganisms from infesting it, that this substance is abiotic or in layman's terms: it is a deadly poison to almost all forms of life.

Trust me, the fish in the sea have fought for millions of years just trying to stay alive while swimming through it – it is a POISON. And you do not need this poison in your body. Therefore, do NOT eat a lot of salt. Sodium by the way is not good for you in overabundance either.

Now remember, just about anything that starts with the name Sodium, Sodium blahblahblahate for example, is SOLUBLE in your stomach. And granted, you actually do need some sodium in your body, what the sports drink people say they give you to replenish your "electrolytes" but you don't need tons of it and potassium and magnesium may be by far the better "electrolytes" over sodium anyway. Also remember that just about anything like blahblahblahium Chloride is also very likely going to be SOLUBLE or EASILY absorbed and also free up the POISON known as CHLORINE. Again, you need a little, so your stomach can actually manufacture the HydroCHLORIC acid it uses to continue your digestive process, but again, you don't need tons of this poison inside of you. Where does the excess of these things go anyway? Straight into the liver.

That's where every single molecule you eat goes by the way, through what the health professionals call affectionately, the HEPATIC PORTAL VEIN. Basically all of the capillaries in the walls of your intestines that are absorbing every molecule of what you ate gather back together into a big vein that feeds directly into your liver. This organ gets the first look at what you had for dinner, every time. This is how what you had for dinner gets regulated. Otherwise you would have dinner, say a steak and a potato, and the potato would be converted into sugars which would hit your bloodstream within an half an hour and you'd be on the same sugar rush as if you had bolted down a two liter bottle of soda – that would not be a very good plan, and so that's why everything funnels into the liver.

The liver will grab up almost everything and then try to slowly release it back into the bloodstream over the next several hours, at least. And in the case of POISONS it does recognize an amazing number of them and tries to permanently take them out of circulation. You can bet it regulates the electrolytes since a particularly salty meal would likely cause you to have a heart attack if it didn't (the electrolytes are involved in the electrical field of the entire human body – subject for a coming book – and dramatically affect the heart which does have a natural pacemaker by the way.) And you can bet it does everything it can, including letting its own cells DIE for the cause, in trying to remove POISONS from the bloodstream coming from the intestines and you can bet that one of these is CHLORINE.

Now the liver can take some abuse along these lines and regenerate on its own, that is its job, but pushing it to its limits and beyond every single day leads to liver disease, liver failure, cirrhosis of the liver (too many cells have been killed repeatedly to the point where it can't grow back as fast as it is being destroyed by the POISON known as ETHANOL – usually – and so the liver literally dies a long slow horrible death and takes the overindulgent drunken idiot through a similar long slow and horrible death along with it.) Yes, you guessed correctly, ETHANOL, the alcohol in alcoholic beverages is one of the worst POISONS you can pickle your liver in – 4 to 6 ounces of alcohol (13% or less) in one sitting one time per day is acceptable for healthy individuals only. Any more than that and you are taxing your liver unnecessarily and that will come back to KILL YOU in the long run.

Ok, so what do we know? Sodium blahblahblahate and blahblahblahium Chloride are both likely very SOLUBLE in our digestive tracts but they will dump unwanted POISONS in the form of excess sodium ions, which the liver will try to regulate, but in the end will release into your blood and remember these are electrolytes and they can really mess up your electrical field and mess with your HEART which is why all the doctors scream – no salt – and the other extremely toxic one CHLORINE which is why they pump the tap water with a fraction of a percent of it which is good enough to kill just about every known microbe on Earth. Microbes are nothing more than single celled organisms … cells … cells that DIE when even a TRACE of CHLORINE is around. Oh yeah, you happen to be made out of cells … cells that die in the presence of chlorine – get it?

Now let's look at a few food label ingredient items shall we? I won't mention the actual food products I found these in, for fear of being mercilessly sued into dust by the greedy money worshipping owners of the companies that manufacture these beautifully packaged POISONS. Here are some of my favorite HORRORS that I have found in food… that you EAT:

1) SODIUM BENZOATE – This may be in every single packaged food product on Earth, or at least in the United States, as a "preservative." Well, it might keep the food the same color and texture for a longer period of time, but it is certainly not preserving the person who eats it. Case in point: Benzene, (the Benzoate ion simply has an oxygen atom bonded to it, which does help lessen its TOXICITY but it certainly does not make it into manna from heaven either) used to be found in every high school chemistry lab in the United States, including my own many years ago. But you won't find it there any more. Why? Because a lab did a study and found that the vapors (it is highly volatile with a unique aroma. Another such small organic molecule with a strange unique aroma is Napthalene or moth balls) and those fumes are extremely carcinogenic and we can't have the children being exposed to

them can we? Absolutely not! But make sure they get their daily DOSE OF THE POISON in the meals they eat EVERY SINGLE DAY! Even if Sodium Benzoate's ion is 1/10,000th the carcinogen as the precursor Benzene, the fact is that every single man, woman and child in the United States eats this POISON almost on a DAILY BASIS. And the last time I checked 300 million divided by ten thousand is still 30,000; as in cases of CANCER. I don't want to be one of them, do you?

2) SODIUM CASEINATE – This is one of my favorites. Ever hear of Casein paint? Basically this food product had wall paint in it and the manufacturer had the audacity to put in parenthesis an explanation for why this ingredient was in the food: "added for texture." They added this garbage – house paint! – to give the food the right TEXTURE. Personally, I think I stopped wanting to eat paint by the time I reached the age of two years old, but thanks anyway.

3) SODIUM STEARATE – Another favorite, this is SOAP. Now I admit I've got quite the potty mouth, but my mother never washed my mouth out with soap, and as an adult I am not about to start either. These monsters didn't even have the decency to explain to me why they put the soap into my food either. Well I guess it keeps it clean right? Ever wonder why soap cleans so well? It bonds with fats and oils and is also soluble in water, this means that it grabs up the oils and dissolves with them into the water and then rinses away squeaky clean. Well I don't want all of my cells which are little bags of water and OIL to get rinsed away leaving my bones squeaky clean ... I'd like to keep all of my cells right there where they are! This stuff is appearing in vitamin pills like crazy as Magnesium Stearate. It is almost impossible to find a pill that does NOT have it. Personally I don't want to swallow a small chunk of soap, but it looks like they are giving us little choice in the matter.

4) YELLOW #5 – This is a particular pet peeve of mine. This well known carcinogen – and I mean there are plenty of studies explicitly showing this nuisance to be a verifiable cancer causing killer – is in almost as many things as that confounded menace Sodium Benzoate. This garbage causes cancer. Do not eat anything containing it and the manufacturers will eventually get the idea and stop using it.

5) The six major SUGAR SUBSTITUTES – acesulfame potassium, aspartame, neotame, sacharrin, sucralose, and sorbitol. I cannot speak for all of them but I can speak for some of them in particular. Saccharin is a well known cancer causing TOXIN; in fact it makes an excellent rat poison and roach killer. Anything that can kill a roach is nothing I want to be eating, these are the critters that can eat book binding glue – get it? Aspartame has some studies linking it to cancer and so does sucralose. I think you're getting the idea: I'd rather risk rotting my teeth than dying of cancer. Now I

know the diabetics are in trouble, they can't just go back to sugar. But that's ok, there are natural sugar substitutes and in their case they may have to consult with a doctor to see which ones will not mess with their blood sugar counts. As for the rest of us, do not bother consuming any artificial sweeteners, they cause cancer, period.

What else can you eat? Go to the meats section and get yourself some chicken, or some fish. I often grab a pack of pork chops when they are on sale. Contrary to popular belief, as long as you cook it well, it won't do any more harm to you in moderation than any other NATURAL thing made by the EARTH as opposed to those things manufactured by some greedy monster. It will certainly do far less harm to me than that little pink packet in your coffee will.

Check the labels. Some brands might add things you don't want. If the chicken looks too yellow, guess what they have bathed it in? Yellow #5, you got it! Incidentally when I indict that garbage I am referring to ALL artificial food colorings and flavors, not just that specific one. Don't eat that POISON.

Yes, I know that most artificial flavorings are chemically "identical" to the real ones found in nature, but why is it that artificial grape flavored things taste nothing like natural grape flavored things? How identical are they? I believe I already warned you about this (sort of the same molecule not being exactly the same) and frankly I do not know how identical these molecules are to the natural ones, and I guarantee you that the greedy monsters POISONING YOUR FOOD with it don't know any more about it than the greatest physicists and chemists on Earth who would neither confirm nor deny my claims with anything more substantial than the Heisenberg Uncertainty principle, which supports my claim that they are different just as much as it would support their claim that undetectable differences are irrelevant. Sorry for the rant, but this stuff is KILLING US and if I get going down hill, there's no stopping me. The bad news is that the greedy monsters putting this manufactured POISONOUS CANCER CAUSING garbage into our food DON'T CARE EITHER. "Just sit down, shut up, buy it and eat it."

Now take a moment to consider the following: how long would you survive without air, in particular oxygen? A few minutes at most. We could therefore say correctly that gaseous oxygen is the ultimate and most essential of all nutrients. Without it a human body shuts down and dies within minutes. This is because the oxygen provides the "oxidizer" for our cells to burn fuel (sugars mostly) from which they derive the energy to function. No energy to function, no life and the main organ that has by far the highest demand for oxygen is the brain and that's exactly why you die so fast without air, because your brain, properly functioning, is that which is conscious and is in essence you. It is fascinating to note that most of the rest of the body can get along quite well for extended periods of time without oxygen, but that is of no use when the brain, which is the person, dies so fast without it.

Now our respiration, our breathing which provides this most essential of all nutrients, only needs to take up oxygen (and get rid of built up Carbon Dioxide which is the result of the metabolic burning of the sugars in our cells) and nothing else; a very simple bodily function and requirement.

The point I am driving at here, is that although the process of eating is not as imperative as breathing, in that you will not starve to death in minutes if you stop (although some people eat as if they think they will) this does not change the fact that if you do stop eating, you will die. Therefore eating is an imperative process, as imperative as breathing, even though the time delay between stopping it is much more protracted, the outcome is the same.

The major difference is that eating which involves the consumption into the digestive tract of essential nutrients, is the opposite of the simplicity of breathing, in which we do it to take up one simple nutrient. In eating, we absorb gigantic collections of gigantic molecules in such profusions and complexities that we may never be able to fully analyze a complete and healthy natural diet consisting of fruits, vegetables, and animal products.

But although we may not be able to fully chemically analyze our nutritional needs, that does not mean that those needs do not exist and it does not mean that we should just throw our hands up and give up. All that this means is that the mad scientists will never be able to provide us with a George Jetson diet of nothing but completely artificially manufactured pills that will keep us healthy for a long lifespan.

What I ultimately want to convince you of, with this argument is that:

1. There can never be an adequate substitution for natural foods. You can certainly take a Vitamin A pill to make sure that you get enough each day, but carrots contain not only all the Vitamin A that you need, but they contain beta-carotene which is a powerful anti-oxidant that helps defend your entire body and all of its cells from being damaged by free radicals or "oxidants" but this exact same substance can be easily converted by the body into more Vitamin A as needed: that's why I would recommend to anyone concerned about Vitamin A to eat carrots, as many as you can choke down, it is very unlikely that you would overdose on beta-carotene although you CAN overdose on pure Vitamin A.
2. By eating natural foods you will take in nutrients that no one even knows exist, but the human body needs them nevertheless. The more variety you have in your natural food diet, the more likely you are to take in something that your body actually desperately needs.

3.   Cravings have been suspected for years to involve a method by which the body reports a serious deficiency to the brain, and the craving is the way in which the brain drives the person to get the missing nutrient. Listen to your cravings and more importantly, keep rotating and changing your diet from one day to the next so that you never fall short for more than five days in a row of anything your body might need.

4.   We know that all of our food, especially in the developed countries, from the plants, fruits, vegetables, grains, to the livestock that feeds on these plants are seriously lacking in critical nutrients because of the long dead dirt in which they have been cultivated. But the grape still looks like a grape, so it has still been able to construct its cells in all of their amazing complexity despite these shortcomings and therefore it has constructed complex molecules, that the mad scientists still have yet to discover or understand, and that your body needs in order to survive and to thrive. So despite my warnings that the plants and animals we eat are deficient, that does not mean that they are devoid of nutritional value. You must eat as many all-natural items in as much variety as you can in order to maintain optimal health and you must avoid at all costs all manufactured and processed foods because they are rife with cancer causing poisons and the processing has destroyed most if not all of the potential nutrients in them.

READING THE INGREDIENTS LABELS

If you do not already know, packaged and processed foods ingredients are listed in order from the ingredient with the highest amount down to the ingredient with the lowest amount in the food. Also, whenever a particular kind of ingredient has been processed in some way, that processing is usually described (only because it is required by either federal law or by enough state laws that the food manufacturers include this additional description so that they can sell their products in all 50 states.)

Here is a typical food ingredients label:

INGREDIENTS: UNBLEACHED ENRICHED WHEAT FLOUR (WHEAT FLOUR, MALTED BARLEY FLOUR, NIACIN, REDUCED IRON, THIAMIN MONONITRATE, RIBOFLAVIN, FOLIC ACID), WATER, HIGH FRUCTOSE CORN SYRUP, CONTAINS LESS THAN 2% OF EACH OF THE FOLLOWING: YEAST, SALT, SOYBEAN OIL, WHEAT GLUTEN, DOUGH CONDITIONERS (CONTAINS ONE OR MORE OF THE FOLLOWING: SODIUM STEAROYL LACTYLATE, MONOGLYCERIDES AND/OR DIGLYCERIDES, CALCIUM PEROXIDE, CALCIUM IODATE, DATEM, ETHOXYLATED MONO AND DIGLYCERIDES, ENZYMES), SOY FLOUR, YEAST FOOD (AMMONIUM SULFATE) , MONOCALCIUM PHOSPHATE, CALCIUM SULFATE, SOY LECITHIN, CALCIUM PROPIONATE (TO RETARD SPOILAGE).

Whew! Where to begin! Well, before we begin could you guess what is in the plastic bag? It's plain, simple, cheap, white bread. I won't mention the brand because it is irrelevant; most white bread ingredients look about the same anyway and there is no sense in "attacking" these people in particular, they all make junk.

Let's break this down, one ingredient at a time:
1. UNBLEACHED ENRICHED WHEAT FLOUR – Well at least they didn't bleach it! So it has retained some trace phytochemicals, but since it is NOT WHOLE GRAIN, the wheat germ has been removed along with MOST of the nutritional value of the wheat kernels. So this is a typical white wheat flour product despite the fact that being unbleached the flour would have been brown.
2. (WHEAT FLOUR, MALTED BARLEY FLOUR, NIACIN, REDUCED IRON, THIAMIN MONONITRATE, RIBOFLAVIN, FOLIC ACID) – This entire list in parentheses behind the first item is the list of the contents of that "unbleached enriched wheat flour." Remember that if they process an ingredient they have to describe it. It looks fairly mundane too. The largest percentage "sub-ingredient" in that flour is wheat flour followed by malted barley flour, then they added niacin (Vitamin B3 because they used the term "enriched" it is the manufactured form) reduced iron (and quite honestly I don't know what that means, but iron is fairly innocuous even if it ends up in the final product as RUST. You just won't be able to absorb most of it, but it won't bother you) thiamin mononitrate which is a manufactured form of Vitamin B1, riboflavin a.k.a. Vitamin B2 (also likely manufactured) and Folic acid a.k.a. Vitamin B9 (this is the ULTIMATE IRONY: by removing the wheat germ – not using whole wheat flour – they felt they had to add the folic acid back in when wheat germ is LOADED with it and of course this is the manufactured form of the vitamin as well as all of the others.)
3, WATER – This is actually the second item in the ingredient list after the unbleached enriched wheat flour because everything in point number 2 above was the ingredient list for that flour. At least they can't screw up water. Oh, I forgot. It could be city pipe water laced with chlorine and fluorine (a known neurotoxin, by the way.)
4. HIGH FRUCTOSE CORN SYRUP – This bane is finding its way into EVERYTHING and it is 100% PURE TRASH CALORIES. And it is the third largest component of the bread after flour and water. Personally, I don't believe they had to try to turn the bread into CANDY. But they did.
5. CONTAINS LESS THAN 2% OF EACH OF THE FOLLOWING: - So from here on out everything in the main ingredients list will be less than 2% of the total mass that went into the oven to be baked. But they do clearly state that there is less than 2% of EACH one of these things, so they can add up to represent a fair percentage of the total mass of the product.

6. YEAST – So up to 2% of the mass that went into the oven was yeast. Well, it is the one that makes the dough become bread rather than a soft wheat flour tortilla.

7. SALT – Since they didn't call it IODIZED SALT, then this is plain and simple salt and the reason I tell people to stay away from packaged and processed foods. They use cheap garbage salt and not the good stuff with the iodine in it. And every bite of packaged and processed trash food is bringing you more and more salt which is an ENEMY of your heart if you do not keep the amount you take in each day under CONTROL.

8. SOYBEAN OIL – I suppose they had to use something in the dough although this is another BANE that is starting to show up in EVERYTHING. Soy beans and ALL of their by-products are NOT HEALTHY FOODS. They have some trace phytochemicals in them that researchers have reported could be detrimental to human health. The cows can eat it but we can't. AVOID ALL SOY BEAN PRODUCTS AND BY-PRODUCTS. They only use it because it is CHEAP and it is also UNHEALTHY GARBAGE.

9. WHEAT GLUTEN – Why they felt they had to add more straight up refined wheat protein is beyond my comprehension but here it is.

10. DOUGH CONDITIONERS – These are the breadmakers "secrets" to making their bread taste better than the other brands.

11. (CONTAINS ONE OR MORE OF THE FOLLOWING: SODIUM STEAROYL LACTYLATE, MONOGLYCERIDES AND/OR DIGLYCERIDES, CALCIUM PEROXIDE, CALCIUM IODATE, DATEM, ETHOXYLATED MONO AND DIGLYCERIDES, ENZYMES), – This list in parentheses following the previous item "dough conditioners" is the list of all of them that they added to the dough. They are mostly MANUFACTURED CHEMICALS of dubious and likely CANCER-CAUSING nature. If it has a name that looks like it should be on the shelf of a chemistry lab, then that is where it should be; NOT IN YOUR FOOD. By the way, that calcium peroxide is BLEACH, so they used unbleached flour, then BLEACHED the whole wad of dough potentially DESTROYING EVERYTHING IN IT ANYWAY. Thanks for nothing.

12. SOY FLOUR – Soy flour is CHEAP GARBAGE FILLER and you should avoid all foods that contain soy or any of its by-products anyway,

13. YEAST FOOD (AMMONIUM SULFATE) – Ammonium sulfate? Come on! Give all the FERTILIZER you want to the yeast, but not me.

14. MONOCALCIUM PHOSPHATE – Not sure why they added CONCRETE (ok, concrete is different, but not by much) I guess they wanted to enrich the bread with calcium in a relatively unusable form and didn't bother to add the vitamin D or any of the other helper nutrients. So instead of giving you stronger healthier

bones and teeth, living on this bread alone will give you kidney stones.

15. CALCIUM SULFATE – a.k.a. Plaster-of-Paris or gypsum. Not sure why they felt the need to put this completely insoluble and un-absorbable garbage into the bread but they did.

16. SOY LECITHIN – Here we go. This GARBAGE (as well as partially hydrogenated or hydrolyzed vegetable oils) is MADNESS. Hydrogenated vegetable oils are basically synthetic animal fat but they contain unusual molecular structures in them that bear the name "trans fats" and these are TOXIC to the liver. I know that some people are suggesting that soy lecithin might even be good for you but it is a cocktail of substances from the soy bean and soy beans are suspected of being problematic so avoid this crud. Lecithin and these hydrogenated and hydrolyzed vegetable oils must be PERMANENTLY PROHIBITED from your house. That my friends is the ONLY WAY they will stop putting this WRETCHED, ACCURSED TRASH into our foods and I am very sure that this bread would be practically the same and a WHOLE LOT HEALTHIER for you without it anyway.

17. CALCIUM PROPIONATE (TO RETARD SPOILAGE) – Just another way to say "artificial preservative." The junk may keep the bread from spoiling but it is certainly not going to do your liver the same favor, instead it will force your liver to absorb it from your food so it doesn't end up in your bloodstream and over time trace chemical additives just like this one can give you liver cancer which is one of the DEADLIEST FORMS OF CANCER known. Do your liver a favor and stop eating POISONS LIKE THIS.

So there you have it. Simple white bread is loaded with TRASH CALORIES when it is completely unnecessary to do that, and it is laced with artificial chemical additives all up and down the ingredients list which are also completely unnecessary. If you want some bread, see if your local bakery will make you some fresh whole grain wheat bread or even rye (it is quite tasty and much better for you anyway.) Also make sure that they do NOT use sodium aluminum carbonate also known as alum in the dough. That is very likely the number one cause of Alzheimer's disease today (many suspect this recent epidemic is caused by chronic trace ALUMINUM poisoning from baking powder and soda cans.)

END OF CHAPTER RECAP

The ingredients you do not want in any of your foods are:

1. Soy beans and their by-products (all cheap garbage fillers)
2. Any manufactured chemicals including but not limited to: artificial colors, flavors, preservatives, sweeteners, and manufactured forms of vitamins and minerals.
3. Processed natural food products like grain flours other than 100% whole grain versions.
4. And absolutely no high fructose corn syrup, no lecithin, and no hydrogenated, or hydrolyzed vegetable oils of any kind.

I know that the previous chapter lists so many bad ingredients in packaged and processed foods that quite literally ALL of them contain at least one item that is so bad for you that it is not worth taking home even if the manufacturer PAID YOU TO BUY IT. The fact that they make us pay for it is downright criminal.

So what's on the menu? All natural whole foods and I know that everything in the produce section has been bathed in pesticides and fungicides (those are the really terrible toxins by the way although many pesticides are just as bad) but I would still rather soak and wash those foods than eat a box of manufactured trash. At least the natural food is bringing a decent share of nutrients in healthy forms as opposed to all of those trash calories and fillers that have about the same nutritional content as the cardboard boxes and plastic bags of their packaging.

The interesting thing about those trace toxins on the produce is that while they too can definitely do harm over the course of decades to the liver in particular, there are many natural phytonutrients that can actually help with that. The chlorophylls in the dark green leafy vegetables (primarily spinach, collard greens, etc.) are excellent detoxifiers and lycopene's potent antioxidant powers also seem to help the liver recover from such damage as well. But you will never get any of these powerful helpers for your body in those cardboard boxes and plastic bags filled with nothing but JUNK CALORIES AND TOXIC CHEMICALS.

THE TOP NUTRIENTS AND THEIR SUPERFOODS

ANTIOXIDANTS – The following are loaded with them: wild blueberries (9,621 ORAC score,) dark chocolate (100% Pure cacao, 20,816,) elderberries (14,697,) cloves (314,446,) cinnamon (267,537,) oregano (159,277,) and turmeric (102,700,) The two best supplements are GLUTATHIONE, and QUERCITIN (Take as directed.) As for Lutein, Vitamin C, astaxanthin, etc. you should definitely get these in their natural whole foods rather than supplements.[42]

FIBER – old-fashioned oatmeal, avocado, artichokes, green peas, acorn squash, Brussels sprouts, chickpeas, lentils, walnuts, apples

All of these are high fiber foods, but in addition to that, most are superfoods that bring either a lot of many essential nutrients (vitamins and minerals) or are the complete source (100% RDA or higher) of at least one essential nutrient.[43]

BETA-CAROTENE – Carrots

Beta-carotene is one of the healthiest phytonutrients on planet Earth. Aside from being the water-soluble and easily absorbed and safely stored form of Vitamin A (straight retinol vitamin A is oil-soluble and the body has trouble handling it in excesses in which it can become toxic) it is also a powerful antioxidant while in this form and has a well studied and verified track record of being very beneficial to many aspects of human health. Carrots are the most readily available source by a large margin and just one medium sized carrot per day brings about 200% of the RDA of beta-carotene as Vitamin A in a perfectly safe form.[1]

LYCOPENE – Tomatoes

Tomatoes are the #1 highest source of lycopene by a wide margin and the lycopene becomes even more available when they are cooked so start making that homemade tomato sauce![2]

ZEAXANTHIN and LUTEIN (often found together) – kale, spinach, turnip greens, collard greens, romaine lettuce, watercress, Swiss chard, mustard greens, yellow and red bell pepper.

Kale has by far the highest concentration of both of these phytonutrients that have been found in significant concentrations in the human eye. Despite the fact that clinical trials with supplements show little effect, these two xanthophylls didn't just magically appear in our eyes and scientists are convinced that we don't manufacture them ourselves. Can't find kale at the store? Spinach or any of the other dark leafy greens will do the trick. Spinach is so loaded up with essential nutrients that a ½ cup raw (4 oz.) in a tossed salad per day is one of my Top Recommended Superfoods.[4]

ASTAXANTHIN (notable mention but found only in a few species of edible red sea algae) – Wild-caught salmon, wild-caught shrimp, crab, lobster

I only included astaxanthin because it happens to be a terpenoid, but it is only found in certain species of oceanic algae and the animals that eat them are LOADED with it. Wild-caught salmon is one of my Top Recommended Superfoods and is loaded with everything from vitamins to minerals to Omega-3 fatty acids and the astaxanthin is what makes its flesh red, so it is by far the most concentrated source of astaxanthin which is one of the most powerful antioxidants known to science. You can't go wrong with wild-caught salmon. Farm-raised salmon are basically starved their entire lives and given a limited selection of foods and the meat is dramatically inferior in all nutrients and it is far less nutritious than wild-caught fish (of any kind by the way.)[6]

OLEANOLIC ACID – olives, olive oil (along with many other phytonutrients unique to olives and olive oil)

Scientists have only begun to scratch the surface with olives and olive oil. This fruit (strange as it sounds it is a fruit by definition despite the unusual taste and characteristics) has several dozen phytonutrients that are unique to it alone and there is plenty of anecdotal evidence and great interest in the scientific community concerning their preventative and curative powers. Go easy on it because although it does contain Omega-6's, and it contains no Omega-3's. If you use it like I do as the ONLY HEALTHY salad dressing (vinegar and oil) then you will need to get a lot of Omega-3 daily to compensate for that.[8]

APIOLE and APIGENIN – Celery

Celery and its close relatives (rhubarb and fennel plant) are loaded with many interesting phytonutrients that are only found in them and there is plenty of preliminary research into these unique phytonutrients that sounds very promising. You can't go wrong snacking on celery during the day since it takes more calories to digest it than it gives you back making it the ultimate dieter's snack food.[20][44]

CARVACROL – oregano, thyme, wild bergamot, savory, marjoram

CARNOSOL – rosemary, sage

While carvacrol is mostly known for its antibacterial properties, carnosol and a few other phytonutrients found in rosemary are under investigation for their anti-carcinogenic properties. So break out those lovely pungent spices and get them into that homemade tomato sauce (amongst other things!)[16]

PERILLYL ALCOHOL – lemongrass, sage, and peppermint

Three fantastic spices that you can grow yourself on a window sill with ease. Add fresh peppermint leaves to your ginger root tea to enhance its flavor and health promoting powers. I dump a tablespoon of sage into my homemade chicken soup along with a large amount of turmeric to make a wonderful broth that turns everything (including the glass lid!) bright yellow and very tasty and healthy too.[12]

LIMONENE – Citrus fruits, marmalades

Most store bought preserves are loaded up with that nightmare high fructose corn syrup making them useless, but all-natural organic orange marmalade will be loaded up with limonene as well as many other interesting phytonutrients like hesperidin. Slather it on anything from French toast to regular whole grain toast for a tasty side dish for breakfast.[45]

VANILLIN (and vanillic acid) - Vanilla bean, traces are found in olive oil, lychee, açaí and cloves. Heating creates traces in coffee, maple syrup, and whole-grain products including corn tortillas and oatmeal.

Vanillin and vanillic acid are only found in natural vanilla extract in significant quantities and although we do not yet know the true extent of their health benefits, I add a few drops to my afternoon coffee to give it a wonderful taste. (Artificial vanilla extract is almost entirely vanillin which is relatively easy to manufacture. Real vanilla extract contains upwards of a HUNDRED different phytochemicals and THAT is the one I believe has many health promoting powers hidden in them all.)[46]

CINNAMIC ACID – Cinnamon, aloe vera.

Cinnamon (all-natural sticks or ground powder) and aloe vera both have extraordinary remedial powers. Cinnamon helps the liver regulate blood sugar and is in my humble opinion

ESSENTIAL to a healthy diet. I dump a load of it onto my French toast or into my morning old-fashioned oatmeal every day for breakfast. I have always suffered from blood sugar issues and I can FEEL the positive effects of that morning blast of cinnamon and I can feel the miserable effects when I skip it too. As for aloe vera, well, I will cover that one in an upcoming volume. I will add volumes to this series and cover several miracle remedial plants per book.[47]

COUMARIN – Citrus fruits.

You simply can't go wrong having a fully ripened grapefruit for breakfast every day. Aside from providing you with a good shot of natural vitamin C, the fruit is loaded with goodies including an enzyme that promotes the burning of fat tissue in the human body (the dieter's number one best friend) and they are loaded with many other interesting and potentially powerful phytonutrients as well. I understand that people on harsh drugs that are MAO Inhibitors are prohibited from eating grapefruits. Do you know why? Because grapefruit contains powerful MAOI's as well – they do the same job as the drug, but are FAR SAFER and FAR HEALTHIER too. I'll eat my grapefruit every morning and never have to take any of those terrible drugs, thank you very much.

PHYTOESTROGENS (large group of compounds; various can be found in) – flax seed, fenugreek, oats, barley, lentils, yams, apples, carrots, pomegranates, wheat germ, coffee, licorice, mint, ginseng, hops (and therefore beer,) fennel, anise.

One of the reasons that researchers are starting to become worried about soybeans and their endless by-products is because they are the number one (highest levels) source of phytoestrogens and in large quantities these can have a negative effect. Don't forget that estrogen is a HORMONE in the human body which means it has powerful and long-term effects on the body. In trace quantities certain phytoestrogens are believed to be very beneficial however and you can see that there are plenty of foods that have various compounds in them. Fenugreek (a spice that I just added to my repertoire) is the source of an extract that is processed into a male fertility product by the way, and it is based on the specific phytoestrogen found in it.[23]

SINIGRIN – broccoli, Brussels sprouts and cabbage.

This and a whole host of other sulfur-containing compounds can be found in these foods. As long as you get enough molybdenum in your daily diet (oatmeal has plenty) then your body will be able to utilize all of that sulfur efficiently and effectively. Sulfur is found in several amino acids and is therefore a component of every protein which is the basic construction material of every cell in your body. Broccoli is one of my Top Recommended Superfoods too.[48]

SAPONINS – Oats, spinach (and other dark leafy greens)

Trace amounts of saponins are believed to enhance digestion and the ability of the intestines to absorb nutrients even though the plant's original goal was to make themselves unpalatable to grazing animals. Apparently they are far more toxic to them (and they do have very different digestive systems compared to ours) than humans. I eat both of these daily, oats for breakfast most days of the week and spinach in my tossed salad for lunch and since I switched to an all-natural whole foods diet I have definitely felt the difference.[7]

RESVERATROL – grapes, raisins, grape juice, wine.

Despite what the scientists and the government are saying (that studies of resveratrol have shown no significant benefits to human health) that does not change the fact that: 1) it is an antioxidant and therefore it must have health promoting powers, 2) It is found in grapes, raisins (best source by the way) grape juice and wine all of which have a litany of other powerful phytonutrients in them as well. The French have always known what they were doing making all of those fine wines! Although there is a definite limit on how much of that you can consume daily, there is no limit on how many raisins you can enjoy. I load up the morning oatmeal with them and snack on them throughout the day. Raisins are a candidate for my Top Recommended Superfoods too.[25]

SALICYLIC ACID – Peppermint, licorice, peanuts and wheat

The active ingredient in aspirin is likely only found in small traces in these regular foods since I never heard anyone suggest eating a peanut butter sandwich to relieve a headache. But ginger/peppermint tea sweetened with honey is incredibly soothing, so maybe the peppermint has enough in it to have a mild effect.[49]

CAPSAICIN – Hot peppers from jalapeno to bhut jolokia

This is the number one plant-based cause of poisoning resulting in emergency room hospital visits in the U.S. I suspect this has to do with idiots trying to prove their manhood by competing in Bhut Jolokia (Indian Ghost Pepper) Eating Contests. And trust me, a few of those will send even the most leather tongued, jalapeño popping fool straight to the emergency room. All kidding aside, too much capsaicin can be a problem not just for the mucus membranes but also for the esophagus, through to the colon. Small quantities however are believed to be beneficial. I am certainly no fool when it comes to hot peppers and I add just a little to my chili, just enough for me to notice that it is there which for most hot pepper enthusiasts would be unnoticeable I guess.[30]

GINGEROL – Ginger root

Ginger is a wonderful spice to cook with and ginger root tea is world-renowned for its powerful remedial properties. Ginger contains a whole array of phytonutrients that are either unique to it, or in vastly higher quantities in it than anything else and I do recommend it on occasion.[31]

ALKYLRESORCINOLS - wheat, rye and barley

I am a huge fan of 100% whole grain breads, but you must still read the ingredients and the makers are still dumping tons of chemical junk into them. You will be far better off getting your bread from a local bakery and rye and barley breads are far tastier and far better for you too.[50]

DITHIOLTHIONES (and ORGANOSULFIDES) – garlic, onions, leeks, chives, and shallots.

These sulfur compounds are of enormous interest to science and have a major impact on human health too. You don't need a lot of them to do the trick either and it seems that nature knows this which is exactly why they are found in foods that we use as spices. I can't load up enough on garlic. It has many potent phytonutrients and is in my Top Recommended Superfoods.[32]

ALLIIN and ALLICIN – garlic

The health benefits of garlic are becoming legendary. Aside from keeping vampires away (and the real ones called mosquitoes too, I am from Florida, I know) garlic is loaded with many interesting substances like these two and all of them are currently under scientific investigation to confirm and identify the exact nature of their many roles in human health.[32]

INDOLE-3-CARBINOL – broccoli, Brussels sprouts, cabbage, mustard greens and kale.

All of these foods are highly recommended and Kale and broccoli are in my Top Recommended Superfoods list for multiple reasons. We might not yet know the full extent of Indole-3-carbinol's health benefits (or many other constituents in the dark leafy greens) yet, but we do know that they are extremely good for you in ways that we do already know about like Vitamin K, Zeaxanthin and Lutein as well as chlorophyll and its powerful detoxification effects which can and does lower the potential for getting cancer and other liver disorders.[34]

ALLYL ISOTHIOCYANATE – horseradish, mustard, and wasabi.

Whether the health benefits of these foods can be attributed to this compound or some other related substance is not yet clear, but we do know that wasabi has a lot of anecdotal claims amongst the Japanese for its health promotional powers. (See the above entry on dithiolthiones.)

PIPERINE – black pepper

Black pepper is definitely on the menu, especially freshly ground peppercorns which also contain traces of capsaicin. (See the above entry on dithiolthiones and capsaicin)

SYN-PROPANETHIAL-S-OXIDE – onions

Onions have endless anecdotal reports on their health benefits ranging from hair growth tonic (doubtful!) to male fertility tonic (possible?) One thing is clear, they are good for you and I include them in everything I prepare from stews to soups to salads. (See the above entry on dithiolthiones)

BETALAINS (group of compounds) – Beets and some are also
found in Swiss chard.

I must admit that even though I loved just about any and all
plant foods I was served as a kid, beets were one of the few I
didn't like very much. But that was then and this is now. Beets are
LOADED with a whole array of phytonutrients either unique to
them are in vastly larger quantities than in any other food source.
Their compounds are relatively uninvestigated too, but that does
not mean that they have no health benefits and I highly
recommend eating them from time to time.[35]

CHLOROPHYLLS – dark green leafy vegetables: spinach,
collards, turnip greens and mustard greens

Now you can see why spinach is in my Top Recommended
Superfoods and the others are excellent for you too.[37]

BETA-SITOSTEROL – vegetable oils, nuts, avocados

This and a whole host of other phytonutrients as well as
essential nutrients are the reason many nuts and avocados are in
the Top Recommended Superfoods list.[14]

MYRICETIN – Most notably found in grapes and wine

Grapes, raisins and grape juice are all Top Recommended
Superfoods because of the vast array of powerful phytonutrients
found almost exclusively in them and nowhere else. Myricetin is
one of the only phytonutrients known that has BOTH antioxidant
as well as oxidant powers meaning that it can give you all of the
classic benefits of antioxidants (relief from oxidative stress in
everything from the eyes and skin, to the heart, to the brain, to the
bones) and can also help combat viral infection. (See the entry for
resveratrol)[18]

CATECHINS (large diverse group) - grapes, raisins, grape juice,
wine, apricots, prune juice, peaches, cocoa, bananas, apples,
apple cider vinegar.

Catechins are a large and diverse group of phytonutrients that
are suspected of having a significant contribution to human
nutrition as well as health. Alone this wouldn't qualify any food for
the Top Recommended Superfoods list, but you can see now why
Grapes, Apricots, Dark chocolate, Bananas and Apples make the
grade.[21]

ANTHOCYANIDINS (large group) - black currants, elderberries,
cranberries, blueberries, blackberries, hawthorn berry,
loganberry, açai, strawberries, (and all of these berry juices,)
red and purple grapes, red wines, cherries, pomegranate (and
the juice,) purple eggplant, black plums, blood oranges, red
cabbage, red and purple onion, purple sweet potatoes, blue
corn, purple and black carrots, red delicious apple

The anthocyanidins are a very powerful class of antioxidants
that are just now starting to get a lot of attention. And while
blueberries make the top of those "Top foods you should never
eat" lists, there are plenty of other foods loaded with them. How do

I get my anthocyanidins? 100% Concord grape juice which is in my Top Recommended Superfoods list.[22]

CURCUMIN – turmeric

While most scientists and profiteers want to convince you that curcumin does no good, I believe they are all lying: the scientists because they can't prove anything with an unstable molecule like curcumin and the profiteers because they can't patent it and make billions off of it. If you don't want to cook with it like I do, take the all-natural supplement. This stuff is very likely a powerful anti-mutagen (prevents and fights cancer.)[26]

INDICAXANTHIN – beets, prickly pear cactus

Although the investigation is in the earliest stages, you can't go wrong eating either food source now and then. The beets are LOADED with several dozen unique compounds and the prickly pear cactus (depends on the species!) is absolutely delicious (ranging from bland to incredibly sweet.)[36]

TANNINS – tea, cocoa

Too many tannins can cause trouble. Most plants have some tannins in them because they serve a wide range of functions in the plants cellular processes. For this reason alone you should get some tannins and Dark chocolate is dark because of the tannins in it and it is one of my Top Recommended Superfoods.[27]

PHYTIC ACID – most grains, nuts, and pumpkin[28]

OXALIC ACID – oranges, spinach, bananas, ginger, almonds, and bell peppers[28]

TARTARIC ACID - apricots, apples, sunflower seeds, avocado, grapes, and tamarind[28]

ANACARDIC ACID – cashews, mango[28]

MALIC ACID – apple

Some of the above unclassified organic acids are under investigation for their potential health benefits. Just like the flavonoids, these contribute to the distinctive flavors of the foods they are in and they could have tremendous health benefits to humans. Most of the foods that have these organic acids in them are already on the menu too.[28]

BETAINE – Wheat, beets

An amino acid prevalent in whole wheat and beets, this constituent of these plant's proteins has shown significant health benefits and it is yet another reason why beets are definitely on the menu. (See Betalains)[39]

OMEGA-6 and OMEGA-3 FATTY ACIDS – vegetable oils, walnuts, chia seeds, flax seeds

Walnuts, chia seeds and flax seeds are the top source of plant Omega-3 ALA (alpha-Linoleic Acid) and are definitely at the top of the list of plant foods you should add to your daily dietary intake. In fact, if you do nothing else with all of the information in this book, do your heart and cardiovascular system a favor and eat ¼ cup of walnuts a day (just 2 ounces) because they will bring you over

2500 mg of Omega-3 and instantly correct your Omega-3 to Omega-6 ratio and go a long way towards lowering and correcting your blood cholesterol levels, improve blood pressure and work to improve your overall cardiovascular health.[40][41]

In the next book I will provide three sections: The Top Recommended Superfoods List and all that each one contains, The complete specific nutrients list and the Top Recommended Superfoods that can provide them (reverse cross reference) and how to read the nutrition labels on our foods.

THANK YOU AND GOD BLESS AND GOOD LUCK AND ABOVE ALL ELSE: TAKE CARE OF YOURSELF (BECAUSE NO ONE ELSE IS GOING TO DO IT)!

REFERENCES

Most information in this book was found at: wikipedia.org, nutritiondata.self.com, myfooddata.com, WebMD, draxe.com, whfoods.com, and the fda.gov and nih.gov. These websites are excellent resources and you should check them out.
[1] https://en.wikipedia.org/wiki/Carotene Retrieved on 08-20-2018
  https://en.wikipedia.org/wiki/Beta-Carotene Retrieved on 08-20-2018
[2] https://draxe.com/lycopene/ Retrieved on 08-20-2018
  https://en.wikipedia.org/wiki/Lycopene Retrieved on 08-20-2018
[3] https://en.wikipedia.org/wiki/Xanthophyll Retrieved on 08-20-2018
[4] https://draxe.com/lutein/ Retrieved on 08-20-2018
  https://en.wikipedia.org/wiki/Zeaxanthin Retrieved on 08-20-2018
[5] https://en.wikipedia.org/wiki/Triterpene Retrieved on 08-20-2018
[6] Rachael Link, MS, RD, https://draxe.com/astaxanthin-benefits/ Retrieved on 08-20-2018
[7] https://en.wikipedia.org/wiki/Saponin Retrieved on 08-20-2018
[8] https://en.wikipedia.org/wiki/Oleanolic_acid Retrieved on 08-20-2018
[9] https://en.wikipedia.org/wiki/Betulinic_acid Retrieved on 08-20-2018
[10] https://en.wikipedia.org/wiki/Diterpene Retrieved on 08-20-2018
[11] https://en.wikipedia.org/wiki/Monoterpene Retrieved on 08-20-2018
[12] https://en.wikipedia.org/wiki/Perillyl_Alcohol Retrieved on 08-20-2018
[13] https://en.wikipedia.org/wiki/Phytosterol Retrieved on 08-20-2018
[14] https://en.wikipedia.org/wiki/Beta-Sitosterol Retrieved on 08-20-2018
[15] https://en.wikipedia.org/wiki/Monophenol Retrieved on 08-20-2018
[16] https://en.wikipedia.org/wiki/Carvacrol Retrieved on 08-20-2018
  https://en.wikipedia.org/wiki/Carnosol Retrieved on 08-20-2018
[17] https://en.wikipedia.org/wiki/Flavonoid Retrieved on 08-20-2018
  https://en.wikipedia.org/wiki/Isoflavonoid Retrieved on 08-20-2018
[18] https://en.wikipedia.org/wiki/Myricetin Retrieved on 08-20-2018
[19] https://en.wikipedia.org/wiki/Hesperidin Retrieved on 08-20-2018
[20] https://en.wikipedia.org/wiki/Apigenin Retrieved on 08-20-2018
[21] https://en.wikipedia.org/wiki/Catechin Retrieved on 08-20-2018
[22] https://draxe.com/anthocyanin/ Retrieved on 08-20-2018
  https://en.wikipedia.org/wiki/Anthocyanidin Retrieved on 08-20-2018
[23] https://en.wikipedia.org/wiki/Phytoestrogen Retrieved on 08-20-2018
[24] https://draxe.com/milk-thistle-benefits/ Retrieved on 08-20-2018
[25] https://draxe.com/all-about-resveratrol/ Retrieved on 08-20-2018
  https://en.wikipedia.org/wiki/Resveratrol Retrieved on 08-20-2018

[26] https://en.wikipedia.org/wiki/Curcumin Retrieved on 08-20-2018
[27] https://en.wikipedia.org/wiki/Tannin Retrieved on 08-20-2018
[28] https://en.wikipedia.org/wiki/Phenolic_acid Retrieved on 08-20-2018
[29] https://en.wikipedia.org/wiki/Hydroxycinnamic_acid Retrieved on 08-20-2018
[30] https://en.wikipedia.org/wiki/Capsaicin Retrieved on 08-20-2018
[31] https://en.wikipedia.org/wiki/Gingerol Retrieved on 08-20-2018
[32] https://en.wikipedia.org/wiki/Glucosinolate Retrieved on 08-20-2018
https://en.wikipedia.org/wiki/Isothiocyanate Retrieved on 08-20-2018
https://en.wikipedia.org/wiki/Indoles Retrieved on 08-20-2018
[33] https://en.wikipedia.org/wiki/List_of_phytochemicals_in_food Retrieved on 08-20-2018
[34] https://en.wikipedia.org/wiki/Indole-3-carbinol Retrieved on 08-20-2018
[35] https://en.wikipedia.org/wiki/Betalain Retrieved on 08-20-2018
[36] https://en.wikipedia.org/wiki/Indicaxanthin Retrieved on 08-20-2018
[37] https://draxe.com/chlorophyll-benefits/ Retrieved on 08-20-2018
https://en.wikipedia.org/wiki/Chlorophyll Retrieved on 08-20-2018
[38] Rohini Nag, https://www.healthkart.com/connect/the-all-essential-amino-acids-foods-list-you-must-know-about/ Retrieved on 08-20-2018
[39] https://draxe.com/what-is-betaine/ Retrieved on 08-20-2018
https://en.wikipedia.org/wiki/Betaine Retrieved on 08-20-2018
[40] https://draxe.com/omega-6/ Retrieved on 08-20-2018
https://en.wikipedia.org/wiki/ Retrieved on 08-20-2018
[41] https://draxe.com/omega-3-benefits-plus-top-10-omega-3-foods-list/ Retrieved on 08-23-2018
https://www.myfooddata.com/articles/high-omega-3-foods.php Retrieved on 08-23-2018
[42] https://draxe.com/top-10-high-antioxidant-foods/ Retrieved on 8-20-2018
http://www.superfoodly.com (ORAC scores) Retrieved on 8-29-2018
[43] https://draxe.com/high-fiber-foods/ Retrieved on 08-20-2018
[44] https://en.wikipedia.org/wiki/Apiole Retrieved on 08-20-2018
[45] https://en.wikipedia.org/wiki/Limonene Retrieved on 08-20-2018
[46] https://en.wikipedia.org/wiki/Vanillin Retrieved on 08-20-2018
[47] https://draxe.com/health-benefits-cinnamon/ Retrieved on 08-29-2018
[48] https://en.wikipedia.org/wiki/Sinigrin Retrieved on 08-20-2018
[49] https://en.wikipedia.org/wiki/Salicylic_acid Retrieved on 08-20-2018
[50] https://en.wikipedia.org/wiki/Alkylresorcinol Retrieved on 08-20-2018
[51] http://www.whfoods.com/genpage.php?tname=nutrient&dbid=128 Retrieved on 08-29-2018
[52] https://en.wikipedia.org/wiki/Chalcanoid Retrieved on 08-20-2018
[53] https://en.wikipedia.org/wiki/Flavonolignan Retrieved on 08-20-2018
[54] https://en.wikipedia.org/wiki/Lignan Retrieved on 08-20-2018
[55] https://en.wikipedia.org/wiki/Stilbenoid Retrieved on 08-20-2018
[56] https://en.wikipedia.org/wiki/Curcuminoid Retrieved on 08-20-2018
[57] https://en.wikipedia.org/wiki/Amine Retrieved on 08-20-2018
[58] https://en.wikipedia.org/wiki/Carbohydrate Retrieved on 08-20-2018
[59] https://en.wikipedia.org/wiki/Protease_Inhibitors Retrieved on 08-20-2018
[60] https://en.wikipedia.org/wiki/Phenylethanoid Retrieved on 08-20-2018

9 781727 101867